HEMODYNAMICS – NEW DIAGNOSTIC AND THERAPEUTIC APPROACHES

Edited by **A. Seda Artis**

Hemodynamics – New Diagnostic and Therapeutic Approaches
Edited by A. Seda Artis

Published by InTech
Janeza Trdine 9, 51000 Rijeka, Croatia

Publishing Process Manager Sasa Leporic

Technical Editor Teodora Smiljanic

Cover Designer InTech Design Team

Additional hard copies can be obtained from orders@intechopen.com

Hemodynamics – New Diagnostic and Therapeutic Approaches, Edited by A. Seda Artis
p. cm.
ISBN 978-953-51-0559-6

For EU product safety concerns:
IN TECH d.o.o., Prolaz Marije Krucifikse Kozulić 3, 51000 Rijeka, Croatia,
info@intechopen.com or visit our website at intechopen.com.

Meet the editor

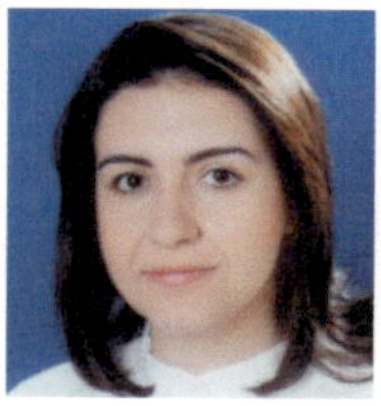

Dr A Seda Artis was graduated from Istanbul University Cerrahpasa School of Medicine, Istanbul, Turkey at 1998. She had experience at different clinics in Turkey and USA as general practitioner or researcher. After completion of her training in Physiology at Erciyes University School of Medicine, Kayseri, Turkey she continued to work at the same place as academic staff. At the moment she is an Assistant Professor of Physiology at Istanbul Medeniyet University School of Medicine, Istanbul, Turkey.

Contents

Preface

Hemodynamics is study of the mechanical and physiologic properties controlling blood pressure and flow through the body. The factors influencing hemodynamics are complex and extensive but include CO, circulating fluid volume, respiration, vascular diameter and resistance, and blood viscosity. Each of these may in turn be influenced by various physiological factors, such as diet, exercise, disease, drugs or alcohol, obesity and excess weight.

A significant majority of all cardiovascular diseases and disorders is related to systemic hemodynamic dysfunction. Hypertension and congestive heart failure are two best known systemic hemodynamic disorders. Also microcirculatory alterations have been repeatedly observed in many physiological conditions and patients with various pathologies such as cardiovascular diseases. To evaluate cardiac functions and peripheral vascular physiologic characteristics hemodynamic monitoring is done. In practice there are both invasive and noninvasive techniques that can be used to determine the hemodynamic status. Generally more severe and more persistent alterations are observed in patients with a poor outcome.

Today many scientists and clinicians are trying to better understand the mechanisms of the hemodynamic changes and to improve the hemodynamic status. So this book is written by expert researchers to address new diagnostic and therapeutic approaches under the scope of hemodynamics.

I wish to thank my family for their support and the authors of each individual chapter for their contribution in summarizing their most relevant findings. I hope that our efforts will not go down the drain.

A. Seda Artis
Physiology Department, School of Medicine,
Istanbul Medeniyet University,
Istanbul,
Turkey

1

The Evaluation of Renal Hemodynamics with Doppler Ultrasonography

Mahir Kaya
Department of Surgery, Faculty of Veterinary Medicine, Atatürk University, Erzurum Turkey

1. Introduction

Gray-scale renal ultrasonography (US) is still performed as a matter of course during the initial evaluation of both native and transplant renal dysfunction. The results, however, often fail to impact on the differential diagnosis or management of renal diseases. Despite major technological advances, gray-scale renal US has remained largely unchanged since the 1970s. It provides only basic anatomical data, such as renal length, cortical thickness, and collecting system dilatation grades. While these may assist in the analysis of disease chronicity, ultrasonographic findings are often normal in spite of the presence of severe renal dysfunction. Clinicians and radiologists are agreed that even the increased renal echogenicity accompanied by renal failure (medical renal disease) requires greater specificity and sensitivity to make it clinically relevant. Collecting system dilatation detection is reliable, though it is not always possible to distinguish between obstructive and non-obstructive pelvicaliectasis on the basis of gray-scale US alone. This purely anatomic approach to renal US, combined with other improved and more economical modalities, has led to nephrologists, internists, and urologists becoming more involved in the field of radiology (Tublin et al., 2003).

Doppler ultrasonographic examination of vascular structures is a fundamental diagnostic technique and one that can also be used to examine organs. Doppler ultrasonographic examination of the kidney, a particularly highly perfused organ, increases the effectiveness of the technique. Color, power and spectral Doppler also supply additional hemodynamics data in addition to the morphological analysis. Renal and extrarenal pathologies as well as other factors also alter renal hemodynamics. Hemodynamic change can be distinguished by variation in intrarenal arterial waveforms. Color Doppler accelerates and facilitates imaging, while duplex Doppler US provides quantitative hemodynamic data. Diseases impacting on organ blood flow may be further characterized by duplex Doppler US. Quantitative Doppler ultrasonographic data include blood flow velocities and volumes. Semi-quantitative data include the indices calculated from blood flow velocities obtained from the spectral Doppler spectrum in renal vessels during the cardiac cycle. These establish resistance to blood flow in the vascular lumen and are a significant source of information about organ perfusion. Three major indices are used in clinical practice: the Systole - Diastole (S/D) ratio, the Pulsatility Index (PI) and the Resistive Index (RI) (also known as the Pourcelot index, resistivity index or resistance index).

S / D = Peak Systolic Velocity / End Diastolic Velocity

PI = (Peak Systolic Velocity - End Diastolic Velocity) / Mean Velocity

RI = (Peak Systolic Velocity - End Diastolic Velocity) / Peak Systolic Velocity

Under normal homeostatic conditions the renal circulation offers low impedance to blood flow throughout the cardiac cycle with continuous antegrade flow during diastole. However, during conditions associated with increased renal vascular resistance, the decrease in renal diastolic blood flow is more pronounced than the decrease in the systolic component. During extreme elevations of renal vascular resistance diastolic flow may be nondetectable or may even show retrograde propagation. Therefore, Doppler ability to characterize altered waveforms in response to elevations of renal vascular resistance may be used to calculate the RI and PI. They were initially introduced for the purpose of determining peripheral vascular diseases. They are also used for the analysis of pathological blood flow patterns and may possibly be used to discriminate among various pathophysiological conditions of the kidney. Resistive index is more widely used than the S/D ratio and PI. Doppler waveform studies are noninvasive, painless, readily available, and relatively easy to perform and learn. Moreover, Doppler ultrasound obviates the need for ionizing radiation and intravenous contrast material administration in situations in which they may be undesirable, such as pregnancy, allergy and renal insufficiency (Rawashdeh et al., 2001).

2. The renal doppler US technique

2.1 Human medicine

The patient has to fast for 8 h prior to the Doppler ultrasonographic examination of the native kidney. The transducer must be positioned so as to visualize the lateral or posterolateral aspect of the kidney. In this position, Doppler examination can be performed with the lowest appropriate angle (0-60^0), establishing an appropriate approach toward vascular structures in the periphery of the hilus and permitting visualization of the kidney without obstruction by gases present in the segments of the intestine and causing artifact. Doppler analysis is then performed.

In intrarenal Doppler ultrasonographic examination, the majority of studies of the potential that have used Doppler US for renal disease evaluation emphasize the importance of applying the most careful technique. It is important to use the highest frequency probe gives that measurable waveforms, with the additional use of color or power Doppler US as appropriate for vessel localization. The arcuate arteries (at the corticomedullary junction) or inter pyelocaliectasic lobar arteries (adjacent to the medullary pyramids) are subsequently insonated with a 2-4 mm Doppler gate. The spectral samples/specimens from the arteries must be analyzed once they have been obtained from three different sites (the cranial, middle and caudal poles). Waveforms should be optimized for measurement by the use of the lowest pulse repetition frequency without aliasing (to maximize waveform size), the highest gain without obscuring background noise, and the lowest degree of wall filter. Three to five reproducible waveforms from each kidney are obtained. Subsequently, the renal Doppler values from these are averaged to establish mean RI and PI values for each kidney.

Once intrarenal Doppler evaluation of the kidney on the investigated side has been completed, the main renal artery and/or veins are analyzed directly. Because of their dimensions, colored Doppler imaging yields no significant contribution to the analysis of these structures, in contrast to intrarenal examination, and gray-scale US is generally employed. However, color Doppler examination is necessary in renal vein thrombosis. The patient is placed in the decubitus or semi-decubitus position, with the kidney to be examined on top, thus permitting transversal visualization of the kidney and including an image of the abdominal aorta. The lateral tip of the transducer is angled slightly toward the caudal aspect, permitting appropriate imaging of the course of the main arterial artery or vein.

It is easier to investigate graft (transplanted) kidneys in the caudal abdomen, located close to the abdominal wall and retroperitoneally, with gray-scale and Doppler US than native kidneys. The hilus must be positioned posteromedially as the transplant kidney is visualized. Gray-scale and intrarenal Doppler evaluations are then performed. Renal artery and vein examination are performed with Doppler mode in the final stage of transplant kidney examination (Platt, 1992; Rawashdeh et al., 2001; Ruggenenti et al., 2001; Tublin et al., 2003; Zubarev, 2001).

2.2 Veterinary medicine

The main renal artery and vein in dogs and cats can be imaged from the hilus of the kidneys as far as their point of origin from the aorta and to the caudal vena cava, respectively. Renal artery diameters are calculated in systole on the basis of gray-scale echo mode. Doppler measurements are performed at the same point (Fig. 1A). In intrarenal Doppler, interlobar branches can be imaged in the proximity of the central echocomplex, since these radiate from the pelvis in the direction of the corticomedullary junction. After branching into arcuate arteries, interlobar arteries flow in the corticomedullary junction. Color Doppler ultrasound can be used to observe the interlobular arteries originating from the arcuate arteries in the cortex. The veins run parallel to the arteries. They are usually wider than the adjacent arteries. The renal arteries exhibit a typical parabolic flow velocity profile (*i.e.*, systolic peaks with broad velocity distribution and no spectral window). The systolic peak is always broad, and it is sometimes possible to observe an *early systolic peak*. Low resistance flow can be determined from a high, continuous diastolic flow, gradually declining during diastole. Following the systolic peak, there is a slight fall in velocity, and then another increase (diastolic peak velocity), gradually decreasing in the rest of the diastole (Fig. 1B). Renal vein flow may exhibit minor changes because of changes in the right atrial and intra-abdominal pressure. An increased forward flow wave follows each heartbeat. If the contractions are in sufficiently close proximity, the next wave (on the Doppler tracing) is superimposed on the previous one, resulting in faster flow. In the event of a more protracted pause between ventricular contractions, the velocity slowly declines in the renal veins superimposed on the previous one, again resulting in faster flow. If the pause between two ventricular contractions is longer, velocity in the renal veins gradually declines; 3.5-7.5 MHz linear or convex transducers can be used. Equipment settings are standardized, and should include a minimum wall filter setting of 50 Hz and a Doppler sample volume between 1 and 3 mm (Szatmari et al., 2001).

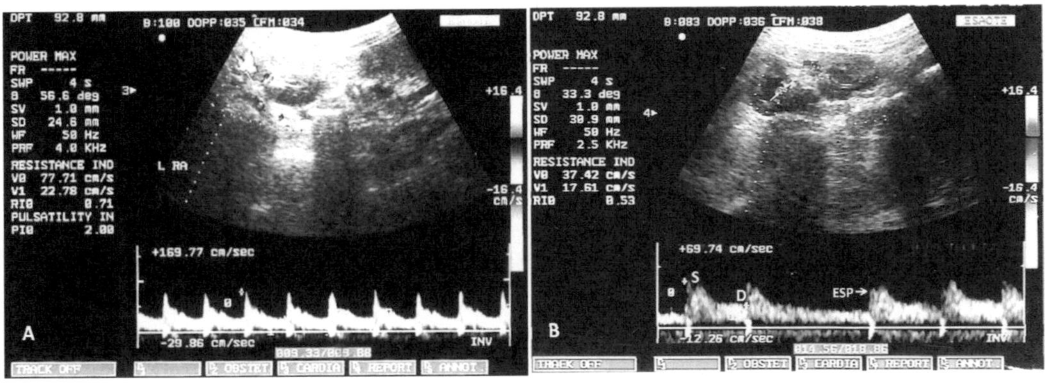

Fig. 1. Duplex Doppler ultrasound images of the left renal artery (A) and the left kidney (B), exhibiting peak systolic blood flow velocity (S), end-diastolic blood flow velocity (D) and *early systolic peak* (ESP) in a healthy dog.

3. Renal resistive index

3.1 Theory

Recent *in vitro* experiments at the University of Michigan have demonstrated the importance of vascular compliance in RI analysis (Tublin et al., 2003, as cited in Bude & Rubin, 1999). Compliance may be defined as the rate of volume change of a vessel as a function of pressure. A pulsating artery expanding in systole and contracting in diastole is a visual manifestation of the effect of compliance. The aim of the *in vitro* experiments was to assess the impact on RI of changes in vascular resistance and compliance. RI was dependent on vascular compliance and resistance. As compliance increased, it became increasingly less dependent on resistance. With zero compliance it was totally independent of vascular resistance. The same team performed another *in vitro* study in which RI decreased with increases in the cross-sectional area of the distal arterial bed. This was again independent from compliance and vascular resistance. Similar *ex vivo* results were produced in a series of experiments from Albany Medical College (Tublin et al., 2003, as cited in Tublin et al., 1999). A pulsatile perfusion system was used to perfuse rabbit kidneys *ex vivo*. Renal vascular resistance, systole, diastole, pulse pressure, and pulse rate were controlled and monitored, while RI was measured simultaneously. A linear relationship was determined between the RI and changes in renal vascular resistance of a pharmacological nature. However, elevation in RI could be related to non-physiological factors that cause in renal vascular resistance. Changes in the RI observed with intense vasoconstriction were only very slightly greater than RI measurement variability. However, RI was significantly affected by alterations in driving pulse pressures. The experiments revealed a linear relationship between RI and the pulse pressure index. The Albany group then performed a series of follow-up *ex vivo* experiments intended to indirectly explore the effect on RI of changes in vascular distensibility (Tublin et al., 2003, as cited in Murphy & Tublin, 2000). They subjected isolated rabbit kidneys to pulsatile perfusion while the renal pelvis was pressurized via the ureter. The team's hypothesis was that subsequent increases in renal interstitial pressure would reduce arterial distensibility and that this would be most apparent during diastole. Arterial distensibility was indirectly assessed on the basis of changes in vascular conductance (flow

/ pressure). They determined that graded increases in renal pelvic pressures led to heightened renal vascular resistance, and that lowered mean conductance led to a higher conductance index (systolic conductance - diastolic conductance / systolic conductance) and increased RI. Their findings emphasize the importance of the interaction among vascular distensibility, resistance, and pulsatile flow in RI analysis. Claudon et al. (1999) replicated many of these findings in a study assessing changes in pig renal blood flow during acute urinary obstruction using contrast-enhanced harmonic sonography. The results of these trials confirm that disease phenomena impacting on vascular distensibility, such as renal artery interstitial fibrosis and vascular stiffening, may also substantially affect the RI.

The unsatisfactory nature of the results obtained using the RI to evaluate ureteral obstruction may perhaps be ascribed to this body of experimental research. The high false-negative rate attendant upon the technique may be due, in some cases, to low-grade, extremely early obstruction or forniceal rupture. At the settings involved and with severe long-standing obstruction, arterial distensibility will only be very slightly affected, since interstitial pressures are relatively normal. The increased reliability of Doppler US in the event of a furosemide challenge being used might also suggest the impact on renal blood flow and the RI of acutely elevated interstitial pressures.

The complex interaction between renal vascular resistance and compliance may also partly account for Doppler US's inability to consistently differentiate types of intrinsic renal disease. It is possible that early reports of elevated RIs with vascular-interstitial disease (but without glomerulopathies) are primarily due to the lower levels of tissue and vascular compliance associated with renal diseases of these kinds (and not only associated with increased renal vascular resistance). Subsequent rather pessimistic reports may also be ascribed to differing patient populations and mixed renal diseases; one isolated RI on its own may not help in the differential diagnosis of intrinsic renal disease because of mixed histology and varying effects on vascular compliance and resistance (Alterini et al., 1996; Pontremoki et al., 1999; Shimizu et al., 2001).

3.2 Resistive index of normal kidneys

3.2.1 Human

3.2.1.1 Adults

A number of studies have cited a value of approximately 0.60 for a normal mean intrarenal RI. The largest series so far (58 patients) reported a mean (± SD) RI of 0.60 ± 0.01 for subjects without pre-existing renal disease (Keogan et al., 1996). Three previous studies cited similar normal mean RI values of 0.64 ± 0.05 (21 patients) (Norris et al. 1984), 0.58 ± 0.05 (109 kidneys) (Platt et al., 1989a), and 0.62 ± 0.04 (28 patients) (Kim et al., 1992). The renal vascular bed in a normal kidney exhibits low blood flow impedance, as reflected by continuous forward flow in diastole in normal adult kidneys (Shokeir et al., 1997a). Most sonographers now regard the upper threshold of the normal intrarenal RI in adults to be 0.70 (Platt et al., 1991a; Platt, 1992).

3.2.1.2 Children and the elderly

Recent studies have shown that mean intrarenal RI is age-dependent, particularly in infants (Kuzmic et al., 2000; Murat et al., 2005; Sigirci et al., 2006; Vade et al., 1993; Wong et al.,

1989). In children, the mean RI frequently exceeds 0.70 during the first year of life. A mean RI of over 0.70 can be observed during the first four years of life at least (Andriani et al., 2001; Bude et al., 1992). In humans, active plasma renin levels are sharply elevated at birth and decrease gradually with age (Fiselier et al., 1984). By 4–8 years, active renin levels exceed those in adults only very slightly. Other renal functional parameters also differ at birth from the corresponding levels in adults. Renal blood flow rate, glomerular filtration rate and tubular excretory capacity for sodium *para*-aminohippuric acid are lower at birth but generally assume adult levels by the age of two. They usually do not mature concurrently. Maturation of renal blood flow rate is, to some extent at least, due to a decrease in renal vascular resistance (Murat et al., 2005). Sigirci et al. (2006) suggested that intrarenal RI was higher for children up to 54 months old than for adults. Therefore, the adult mean intrarenal RI criterion of 0.70 should be applicable to children 54 months old and older. The age dependency of the intrarenal RI is directly related to that of plasma renin and aldosterone levels in healthy children whom Doppler parameters and blood analysis are evaluated synchronously.

The intrarenal RI values in patients aged over 60 tend to be higher than those in younger adults (Rawashdeh et al., 2001; Terry et al., 1992). This may be ascribed to true renal dysfunction in senescent kidneys and that is not solely due to misleading variations or an age-dependent variability in the RI (Platt et al., 1994a). This suggestion is based on the fact that elevated values in patients over 60 are correlated with compromised creatinine clearance. Another study demonstrated that average RI levels increases by 0.002 on an annual basis (Keogan et al., 1996). This is possibly due to a progressive decrease per decade of some 10%, the result of functional and anatomical changes in the renal vasculature with increasing age (Rawashdeh et al., 2001).

3.2.2 Animals

In a study involving 20 healthy young pigs, Rawashdeh et al. (2000) demonstrated a normal RI range of 0.48 to 0.85 (0.63 ± 0.09). Pope et al. (1996) reported a 95% confidence interval (CI) from 0.43 to 0.63 (0.53 ± 0.05) in another porcine study. Baseline values in studies on rabbits vary between 0.51 ± 0.04 and 0.54 ± 0.11 (Chu et al., 2011; Kaya et al., 2010; Kaya et al., 2011). An intrarenal RI range of 0.52 - 0.73 have been reported for healthy dogs (Nyland et al., 1993), and of 0.44 – 0.71 for healthy cats (Rivers et al., 1996). Another study reported an intrarenal RI was 0.61 ± 0.06 in 22 normal kidneys in dogs (Morrow et al., 1996). In 11 mongrel dogs, the RI range was 0.54 to 0.75 (0.64 ± 0.05) (Dodd et al., 1991a). However, Ulrich et al. (1995) reported a 95% CI of 0.46 - 0.62 (0.54 ± 0.04) in six mongrel dogs. In a study of healthy Persian cats, main renal artery RI values for the right kidney were 0.52 ± 0.07 and 0.55 ± 0.07 for the left kidney, with an intrarenal RI value obtained from the interlobar arteries of 0.51± 0.07 (Carvalho & Chammas, 2011). Another study reported intrarenal RI values for normal cats as 0.59 ± 0.05 for the right kidney and 0.56 ± 0.06 for the left kidney, with no statistically significant differences observed between them (Nyland et al., 1993). In another study, intrarenal RI values for mixed-breed cats were 0.61 ± 0.04, and 0.60 ± 0.07 for Turkish angora cats (Gonul et al., 2011). There is no considerable difference among breeds, but species. Such findings may simply reflect the varied nature of the species and breed studies' inherent physiological qualities (Rawashdeh et al., 2001). Renal dimensions and intrarenal RI have been correlated to the body weight of cats (Park et al., 2008). Studies comping with the age-intrarenal RI relationship and renin–angiotension–

aldosterone system are limited. Mechanism by renin–angiotension–aldosterone system plays a role has not been clearly established in dogs and its effect in clinic application is not yet completely understood. In a study by Chang et al. (2010), the intrarenal RI in dogs younger than 4 months was higher than in older dogs. Therefore, the use of 0.73 as the upper limit for intrarenal RI in normal dogs is not appropriate for dogs younger than 4 months. They also stated that plasma renin activity was an important factor in the age dependency of the RI in dogs <4 months of age (Chang et al., 2010).

An elevation in the mean intrarenal RI (>0.70) has been determined for the clinical diagnosis of canine acute renal failure and congenital dysplasia. Considering RI greater than 0.70 abnormal, the sensitivity and specificity of the RI in differentiating between normal and abnormal kidneys were shown to be 38 and 96%, respectively (Morrow et al., 1996). When vascular resistance rises, diastolic blood flow is reduced to a greater degree than systolic blood flow (Rifkin et al., 1987). The relatively greater decrease in end diastolic velocity compared to peak systolic velocity then causes an elevation in RI and PI. The upper threshold for RI and PI need to be established in order to identify an abnormally increased vascular resistance. There are slight differences in the upper threshold (calculated as means + 2 standard deviations) for RI between various studies. Some suggest an upper value of 0.70 for cats and dogs (Morrow et al., 1996; Rivers et al., 1996). This is the same value as that proposed as a limit for normal mean intrarenal RI in humans. Other studies have suggested an upper value of 0.73 for dogs and 0.71 for cats (Nyland et al., 1993; Rivers et al., 1997a).

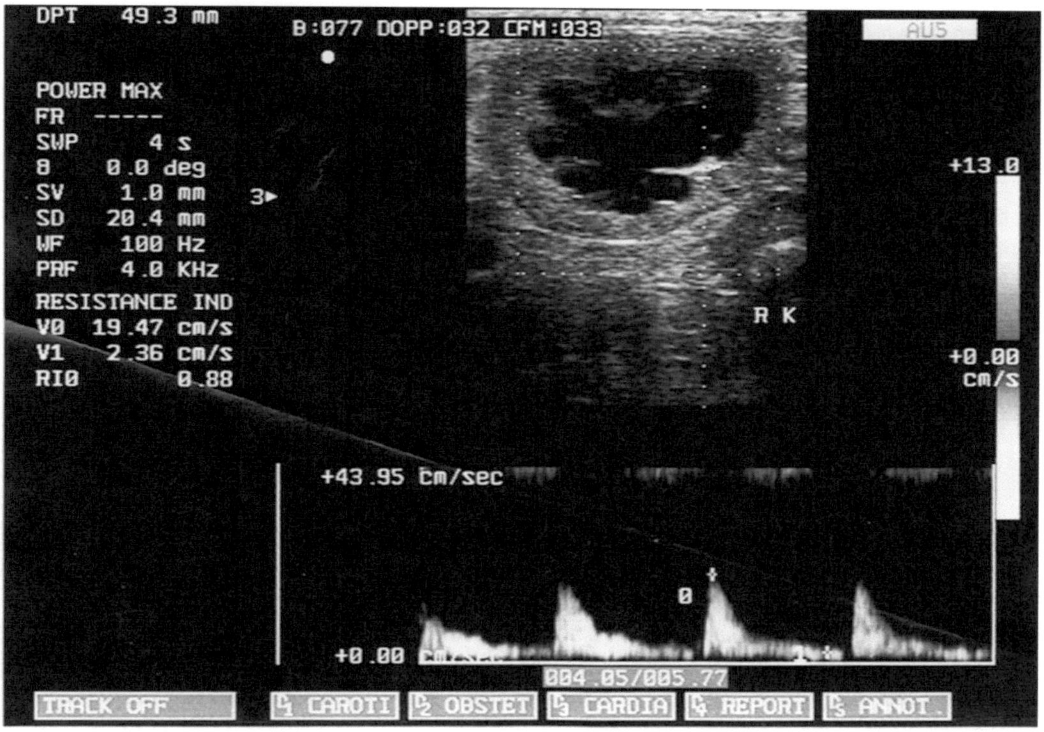

Fig. 2. Duplex Doppler ultrasound image of hydronephrotic kidney developed after the right ureter ligation in an ovariohysterectomized cat. Increased intrarenal RI (0.88) in intrarenal arterial flow pattern is shown.

Novellas et al. (2007) suggested a similar upper threshold for the RI of 0.72 for dogs and 0.70 for cats (Fig. 2.). The same study suggests an upper level for intrarenal PI of 1.52 in dogs and 1.29 in cats. However, an earlier study suggested a mean intrarenal PI value of 0.80 ± 0.13 (Morrow et al., 1996) and emphasized that the upper threshold value should be 1.06 (Novellas et al., 2007). However, no sensitivity and specificity were reported in these studies.

4. Factors affecting renal resistive index

4.1 Pulse and blood pressure

Tublin et al. (1999) reported a significant direct linear relationship between intrarenal RI and pulse pressure. This suggests that RI increases in line with the widening of the pressure difference between systole and diastole. In the event of an elevated RI being observed in a patient with presumed normal kidneys, the data should be correlated with the patient's heart rate and blood pressure. Heart rate and blood pressure at physiological extremes can alter the intrarenal RI without renal pathology being present. It is therefore important to establish these two variables in order to interpret the intrarenal RI accurately. Significant hypotension and a low heart rate can produce an elevation of RI without a true change in renal vascular impedance (Mostbeck et al., 1990). Hypotension reduces diastolic volume in the spectrum. This, in turn, leads to a significant elevation in RI value. Bradycardia and hypertension also lead to elevated intrarenal RI. If blood pressure and heart flow are stable, an increase in heart level causes intrarenal RI to fall. Tachycardia also leads to a fall in intrarenal RI (Shokeir et al., 1997a).

4.2 Dehydration

The intrarenal RI values ≥0.70 have been reported in 54% of non-obstructed kidneys in fasting children. The intrarenal RI resumes its normal value after hydration, indicating the importance of oral hydration at least for the proper interpretation of Doppler studies (Shokeir et al., 1996, 1997a).

4.3 Anesthesia

Doppler US is used in human medicine to determine blood flow without sedation. However, sedation may be required prior to imaging in veterinary medicine for purposes of restraint because poor patient cooperation, high respiratory and heart rates and voluntary movement may interfere with the outcome, particularly in cases involving detailed investigation, such as abdominal vascular US. Anesthetic agents may change systemic and renal hemodynamics and subsequently impact on vascular resistance. Extensive data on the cardiovascular effects of drugs can be obtained through Doppler flow technology using high-resolution vessel images together with hemodynamic monitoring. A combination of atropine, diazepam, acepromazine, and ketamine has been shown to reduce the intrarenal RI in healthy dogs (Rivers et al., 1997b). Sedation with a combination of atropine, acepromazine, and ketamine did not alter the intrarenal RI in cats (Rivers et al., 1996). Yet, anesthesia with isofluorane did increase both the intrarenal RI and PI in cats (Mitchell et al., 1998). In one study coping with the effects of short-term anesthetics on renal hemodynamics it was shown that while propofol had a minimal effect, a xylazine-ketamine combination and thiopental caused a significant drop in intrarenal RI (Kaya et al., 2011).

4.4 Extrarenal factors

The effect of vascular compliance on RI may account for the positive nature of studies investigating the usefulness of Doppler US in assessing end-organ damage in patients with hypertension and arteriosclerosis. Several recent studies showed that an elevated RI was correlated with left ventricular hypertrophy and carotid intimal thickening (Alterini et al., 1996; Pontremoki et al., 1999; Shimizu et al., 2001). Studies have also identified compression as an extraneous factor capable of elevating intrarenal RI. Compression may result from the effects of hematoma or another lesion occupying space and exerting pressure in the area surrounding the kidney. Subcapsular or perinephric fluid collection has also been associated with increased intrarenal RI in humans. Manual compression transmitted through the ultrasound transducer may lead to false iatrogenic increases in intrarenal RI, as well (Pozniak et al., 1988).

4.5 Renal medical diseases

Nephrologists and radiologists have long been frustrated by the lack of specificity inherent in gray-scale examination in evaluating intrinsic renal disease. Although renal size, cortical thickness, and echogenicity may be helpful in assessing disease chronicity, these are typically of no assistance in the differential diagnosis or management of renal disease. Doppler US possibly being able to serve as a useful adjunct for the gray-scale assessment of renal disease was proposed in a series of papers by the University of Michigan team. In Platt et al. (1990)'s preliminary research, 41 patients' renal biopsy results were correlated with RI analysis. In this study, normal RI values were determined in patients with isolated glomerular disease (mean, 0.58), whereas subjects with vascular or interstitial disease had significantly elevated RI values (means, 0.87 and 0.75, respectively).

Patriquin et al. (1989) reported an elevated RI during the anuric-oliguric phase of acute renal failure in 17 children. Intrarenal RI has also been thought to exhibit strong correlation with renal involvement in progressive systemic sclerosis (Aikimbaev et al., 2001). Hepatorenal failure is a well-known complication associated with established liver disease. It is characterized by early renal hemodynamic changes (vasoconstriction) prior to clinically recognized kidney disease. It should be possible to detect this renal vasoconstruction (increased renal vascular resistance) noninvasively by the use of Doppler US. It is also possible to identify nonazotemic patients with liver disease, a subgroup at significantly greater risk for subsequent kidney dysfunction and the hepatorenal syndrome using renal duplex Doppler US (Platt et al., 1994b). Doppler US's ability to identify latent hepatorenal syndrome before liver transplantation was again demonstrated by the University of Michigan group (Platt et al., 1992). Doppler US was useful outcome predictor in patients with lupus nephritis: an elevated RI value was shown to predict poor renal outcome in a prospective series involving 34 patients with various degrees of nephritis, including in subjects with normal baseline renal functions (Platt et al., 1997). Doppler US has also been proposed as a useful tool for the analysis of non-obstructive acute renal failure; an RI greater than 0.07 was determined as a reliable discriminator between acute tubular necrosis and prerenal failure (Platt et al., 1991b). Diabetes also affects intrarenal RI values; intrarenal RI is particularly elevated in established diabetic nephropathy. The intrarenal RI may actually fall to levels significantly below normal during the early stages of preclinical diabetic nephropathy, which is probably associated with the state of decreased renal vascular resistance accompanying preglomerular vasodilatation in the early stages of diabetic kidney involvement (Derchi et al., 1994; Platt et al., 1994a). The intrarenal RI has also found adherents as a useful marker of diabetic nephropathy (Frauchiger et al., 2000; Soldo et al., 1997). In contrast, other studies have suggested that Doppler US provides little more than serum creatinine levels and creatinine clearance rates in patients with early diabetic nephropathy and normal renal functions (Marzano et al., 1998; Okten et al., 1999; Sari et al., 1999). The intrarenal RI is significantly greater in pregnant patients with pyelonephritis than in pregnant women without pyelonephritis (Keogan et al., 1996b). Biopsy correlated studies have verified these findings and assessed the role of the intrarenal RI for differentiating among various renal medical diseases with encouraging results (Platt et al., 1990; Platt et al., 1991b). Therefore, it may be difficult to diagnose unilateral obstruction in patients with a known renal medical condition. However, renal medical disease is usually a bilateral symmetrical affliction (Rawashdeh et al., 2001).

Earlier studies reported elevated renal vascular impedance with chronic hypertension (Norris et al., 1989) and acute renal failure (Wong et al., 1989). The intrarenal PI and RI would appear to be closely related to renal hemodynamic parameters and creatinine clearance in patients with chronic renal failure and hypertension (Petersen et al., 1995). Platt et al. (1989b) found elevated intrarenal RI in half of 50 patients with renal medical diseases. An elevated intrarenal RI could therefore be due to renal disease or obstruction, in the context of known medical renal disease and pyelocaliectasis, thus limiting the value of an abnormal intrarenal RI in this particular situation.

In a dog with acute tubular necrosis intrarenal RI values were observed to be greater than 0.73, normalizing after effective treatment (Daley et al., 1994). One retrospective study investigated intrarenal RI levels in 67 dogs with spontaneous non-obstructive renal disease. Histopathological or cytological findings were present in 12 of these, four of which had tubulointerstitial disease with or without glomerular disease, and three had glomerular disease alone. Three of the four dogs with tubulointerstitial disease had intrarenal values greater than 0.73, while lower values were observed in the three animals with glomerular disease alone. The authors suggested that increased intrarenal RI was compatible with tubulointerstitial, as opposed to glomerular disease (Marrow et al., 1996). In our clinical observations, intrarenal RI may increase in dogs with pyelonephritis (Fig. 3.). The correlation between serum creatinine concentration and intrarenal RI in humans is positive, but weak. Proteinuria has not been associated with increased intrarenal RI in humans (Platt et al., 1990, Platt 1992). Similarly, no statistically significant correlation between individual dog and cat intrarenal RI and serum creatinine concentration was determined. Neither was any statistically significant correlation identified between individual dog intrarenal RI and urine protein-to-creatinine ratio in that study. Intrarenal RI values broadly overlapped compared with urine output in cats with non-obstructive renal disease. The sensitivity was reported to be 57%in dogs with increased intrarenal RI in determining non-obstructive renal disease (tubulointerstitial or glomerular disease) (Rivers et al., 1997a). Another study reported a sensitivity of 38% for increased intrarenal RI (>0.70) in the detection of non-obstructive renal disease in 67 dogs. Sensitivity of 90% has been reported for increased intrarenal RI in the determination of non-obstructive renal disease in azotemic cats. Increased intrarenal RI has a 40% level of detection of renal obstruction in cats with pelvicoureteral dilation during gray-scale US (Morrow et al., 1996). Increased intrarenal RI in dogs and cats with higher relative renal cortex echogenicity may be the result of renal disease, as opposed to normal variation; further studies involving clinicopathological analysis of such subjects are now required. Increased intrarenal RI values observed in azotemic dogs with spontaneous non-obstructive renal disease are probably associated with active tubulointerstitial, as opposed to glomerular disease. However, increased intrarenal RI alone does not rule out the presence of glomerular disease. Renal Doppler evaluation of intrarenal RI is useful as an ancillary diagnostic technique in azotemic dogs and cats with non-obstructive renal disease. This is particularly the case when gray-scale US findings are not definitive. Increased intrarenal RI can only be of restricted use in evaluating the severity of concurrent renal dysfunction. Intrarenal RI may subsequently return to normal following the administration of appropriate treatment in dogs with non-obstructive renal disease and in cats with both non-obstructive and obstructive disease (Rivers et al., 1997a).

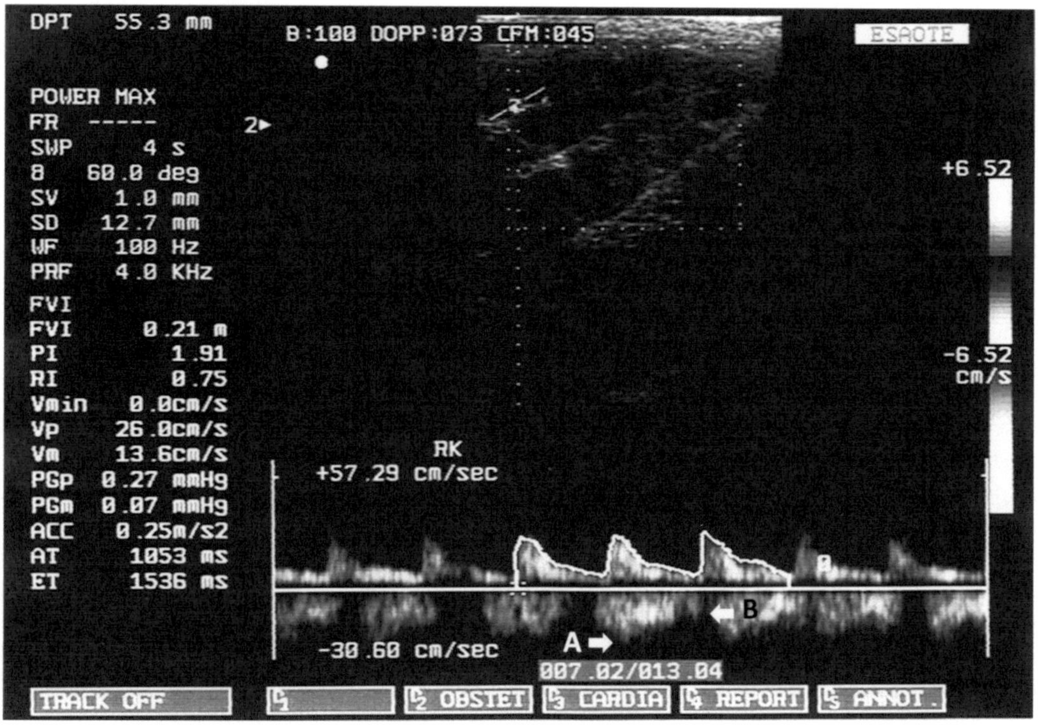

Fig. 3. Arterial and venous flow patterns in the right kidney of a dog with acute pyelonephritis. The peak venous flow signal (A) and the least flow signal (B), used in intrarenal venous impedance index, as well as elevated intrarenal arterial indexes are shown.

4.6 Renal neoplasias

Renal Doppler US does not contribute anything to gray-scale US in the diagnosis of simple cysts representing the great majority of renal masses. In contrast, the blood flow spectrum cannot be determined in septum cysts or in the presence of other solid components using Doppler US. In malign renal neoplasias, a high-velocity and low-resistance arterial flow spectrum associated with the hemodynamic characteristics of neovascularization originating from arteriovenous relations and the high pressure difference caused by them can be observed. In benign neoplasia, on the other hand, no specific and measurable Doppler flow spectrum has been reported. Blood flow velocities similar to those in the abdominal aorta were reported in blood flow specimens obtained from renal cell carcinomas. Malign renal neoplasia, and particularly renal cell carcinoma, exhibit vascular and especially venous invasion. Thrombus in the renal vein or lumen of the inferior vena cava prevents the formation of blood flow-associated colorization. In contrast to benign hemorrhagic thrombus, blood flow signals can be determined by Doppler US in neoplastic thrombus. When the renal vein is completely obstructed by thrombosis, the finding to be determined with Doppler US is low, zero or below baseline diastolic volume in the intrarenal arterial structures, in other words, elevated blood flow. Renal Doppler US is also useful in the evaluation of masses inside the collecting system, such as renal parenchymal masses. Determination of the vascular flow spectrum or Doppler signals obtained from such neoplasia tumoral masses permits differentiation of non-neoplasia lesions such as coagulum or debris, from collecting system neoplasias. However, Doppler signals may not be observed in cases of deep localization or in which the lesions are small, or because the device or transducer are not set at the optimal level (Kier et al., 1990; Ramos et al., 1988).

5. Renal pathologies affecting renal hemodynamics

5.1 Renal vascular pathologies

5.1.1 Renal artery stenosis and occlusion

Renal artery stenosis is most commonly caused by either fibromuscular dysplasia or atherosclerosis. It may develop alone or in association with hypertension, renal insufficiency (ischemic nephropathy), or both. As a cause of hypertension and renal ischemia, renal artery stenosis resulting from atherosclerotic changes in the renal artery is now a serious concern, as it often leads to end-stage renal failure (Scoble, 1999). Hemodynamically, significant narrowing of the renal artery (a decrease in renal artery diameter ≥ 60%) leads to treatable hypertension. Since renal angiography is invasive and requires the use of contrast material, it is not widely used. In recent years, research has been focused on non-invasive diagnostic techniques, which might reliably predict the outcome of blood pressure and renal function after revascularization of renal artery stenosis. Renal artery stenosis is one of the most frequent indications for renal Doppler ultrasonographic examination, and renal Doppler US with a considerable reliability has been used in the diagnosis of renal artery stenosis and occlusion since 1984 (Avasthi et al., 1984).

An elevated flow rate is one of the hemodynamic findings in renal artery stenosis. Studies have shown that blood flow velocity is greater in the point of stenosis than normal renal artery velocities. In addition to blood flow velocity, turbulence in the blood flow spectrum post-stenosis is another important finding. The first studies regarded a blood flow velocity of 100 cm/s as the upper limit, while later research suggested the limit should be 170 - 200 cm/s. In these studies sensitivity was 81% - 92% and specificity was 87% - 96% (Gottlieb et al., 1995; House et al., 1999; Krumme et al., 1996; Miralles et al., 1996). However, the renal-aortic ratio obtained by dividing the renal artery flow velocity by the abdominal aorta flow velocity can be used to eliminate individual differences. A level ≥3.5 is regarded as diagnostic for renal artery stenosis, and has a sensitivity of 92% and specificity of 76% in renal artery stenosis diagnosis (Miralles et al., 1996). Various factors, such as the experience of the physician performing the examination, patient cooperation, meteorism and obesity improve the practicality of the technique. Because of these limitations, technical imaging is easier in the diagnosis of renal artery stenosis, hemodynamic changes in the intrarenal arteries are used. Changes in the acceleration parameters of the blood flow spectra obtained from the level of the renal hilus can be used in the diagnosis of renal artery stenosis. Accordingly, a delayed rise in peak systolic velocity, low flow velocity and a blunt peak (pulsus tardus et parvus) and renal hemodynamic change in this vascular pathology make the Doppler spectrum diagnostically important (Handa et al., 1986). Intrarenal Doppler parameters such as decreased flow velocity, low RI (<0.50) and PI values, decreased acceleration (<3 m/s^2) and increased acceleration time (>70 m/s) are also considered in renal artery stenosis (Bude and Rubin 1995). Comparison of intrarenal RI and PI values on the side with pathology with the contralateral kidney also improves diagnostic success in unilateral renal artery stenosis (Krumme et al., 1996; Riehl et al., 1997). Another study suggested that the normal early systolic peak that should normally be observed disappears (Stavros et al., 1992). The sensitivity of intrarenal Doppler parameters declines in cases with high vascular resistance (RI > 0.70) (Stavros & Harshfield, 1994). Renal Doppler indices return to normal following treatment of renal artery stenosis (Ozbek et al., 1993). When renal artery and intrarenal Doppler parameters are considered together, sensitivity in the diagnosis of renal artery stenosis is 89%, and specificity of 92% (Krumme et al., 1996).

Various renal pathologies, such as atherosclerosis, and trauma or iatrogenic causes may lead to renal artery occlusion. In renal artery occlusions exhibiting acute development or with insufficient collateralization, blood flow in the renal arteries cannot be imaged with color or power Doppler, and the Doppler spectrum cannot be determined. At the same time, either a very weak blood flow spectrum is obtained from the intrarenal arteries, or else arterial flow cannot be established at all. For these reasons, the use of ultrasonographic contrast material in the diagnosis of renal artery stenosis enhances the success of renal Doppler US. The ultrasonographic contrast materials may make it easier to distinguish the renal arteries by increasing the Doppler signal intensity and that the inadequacy stemming from the inability to identify these arteries can thus be eliminated. Claudon et al. (2000) reported the sufficient investigation level rose from 64 to 84% with the use of ultrasonographic contrast material. Missouris et al. (1996) reported that with the use of SH U 508 A (Levovist ®), sensitivity in diagnosis of renal artery stenosis rose from 85 to 94%, and specificity from 79 to 88%. At the same time, while a shortening in investigation time has been reported with the use of these contrast materials, the high price of ultrasonographic contrast materials means they are not economical. Moreover, ultrasonographic contrast materials make a positive contribution in the presence and evaluation of accessory arteries, which represent a significant limitation in renal Doppler ultrasonographic examination and levels of observation of renal artery stenosis rose to 77% (Melany et al., 1997).

5.1.2 Renal vein thrombosis

Renal vein thrombosis is a known cause and complication of renal diseases. The acute form of this vascular pathology may arise in association with such causes as sudden water loss, hypercoagulopathies, trauma, malignity and sepsis in children. One specific finding in gray-scale ultrasonographic examination of renal vein thrombosis is an increased thickness in renal parenchymal thickness. Decreased echogenicity in the renal cortex or a heterogeneous appearance observed together with cystic areas are other findings determined in gray-scale US. Increased renal cortex echogenicity is a finding that can appear in advance stages of pathology. Despite not being specific, increased dimension in the renal vein is regarded as a non-specific finding. Thrombus inside the vein can be monitored in this pathology using gray-scale US. No blood flow findings being determined at renal Doppler US is sufficient for a diagnosis of renal vein thrombosis. Blood flow in the renal vein however may not be to established due to faulty devices or settings. All device settings must therefore be optimal for diagnosis. In addition, factors such as collapse of the renal vein due to inappropriate Doppler angle or probe pressure or blood flow being too decreased to measure due to valsalva can also have a negative impact on flow hemodynamics obtained from the renal vein. In cases in which no results can be obtained from Doppler examination of the renal vein, for reasons such as obesity or meteorism or in which direct imaging needs to be supported, intrarenal Doppler examinations can be performed. Elevated flow resistance is noteworthy among the intrarenal Doppler US findings for acute renal vein thrombosis. This develops in association with insufficient venous drainage and/or intrarenal edema. This, in turn, leads to high intrarenal RI and PI values. With a decrease in diastolic flow component, or it being below the baseline, forward and backward blood flow specimens may arise in the Doppler spectrum. These findings may lose specificity as a result of venous collaterals, such as capsular veins in the native kidney, becoming involved. Diagnosis of chronic renal vein thrombosis is more difficult than that of acute renal vein thrombosis. As with acute renal vein thrombosis, the observation of thrombus inside the vein at gray-scale US, or no or only partial blood flow findings from Doppler US can establish pathology. However, the kidney and renal vein frequently being normal size and intrarenal Doppler findings not emerging due to collateralization are factors complicating the diagnosis of chronic renal vein thrombosis (Chen et al., 1998; Helenon et al., 1995; Zubarev, 2001)

5.1.3 Arteriovenous fistulas

Renal arteriovenous fistulas frequently arise as a result of renal biopsy or other medical procedures. Renal Doppler US is quite successful in determining this pathology. Arteriovenous fistulas of clinically insignificant size may even be identified in a noninvasive form as a result of hemodynamic effects established by renal arteriovenous fistulas. High velocity flow at the fistula level, a consequent color artifact in the surrounding tissue, high-velocity and low-resistance arterial flow in the artery, and high-velocity and pulsatile (observed with arterial spectrum) flow in the vein are some Doppler US findings of arteriovenous fistulas. The focus of the high blood flow velocities determined from the level of the arteriovenous fistula itself is a prominent finding (Helenon et al., 1995; Ozbek et al., 1995). In color Doppler, adjustment of the color filter to high velocities and the elimination of low velocities facilitate the diagnosis of arteriovenous fistulas (Edwards & Beggs 1987).

5.1.4 Aneurism and pseudoaneurism

Renal arterial aneurisms can easily be diagnosed in cases where the lesion is determined with gray-scale ultrasound. A Doppler wave form is determined within the cystic structure identified. Like arteriovenous fistulas, pseudoaneurisms are frequently of iatrogenic origin and generally co-exist. Pseudoaneurisms are generally seen as cystic cavities within the renal parenchyma that cause an arterial spectrum at Doppler analysis. Cystic structures may gradually thrombose, either partly or completely (Chen et al., 1998; Zubarev, 2001).

5.2 Ureteral obstruction (obstructive uropathy)

Ureteral obstruction is one of the most important pathologies of the urinary system. Caused by a number of factors, it may lead to kidney failure and is characterized by irreversible and reversible destruction in the kidneys and ureter. Etiological factors include congenital, acquired, and predisposing elements. As well as distinguishing between obstructive and non-obstructive dilatation, the localization and extent of the obstructed area must also be determined in order to avoid unnecessary surgery. The early diagnosis and release of obstruction are essential if irreversible damage in the affected kidneys is to be prevented. Various imaging methods are used in the diagnosis of ureteral obstruction, including radiography, excretory urography, gray-scale US, Doppler US, computed tomography, magnetic resonance imaging and percutaneous antegrade pyelography. The majority of studies regarding renal Doppler US have concentrated the potential role of Doppler US in evaluating ureteral obstruction.

5.2.1 Complete obstruction

Gray-scale examination for potential acute and chronic obstruction has been known to have attendant limitations since the mid-'80s. Ultrasonography provides purely anatomical data, and these may be incomplete or absent: non-obstructive conditions (residual dilatation from previously existing relieved obstruction, pyelonephritis, congenital malformation, reflux and diuresis) may also give rise to collecting system dilatation. While conventional gray-scale US only supplies an anatomical image of the changes (e.g., pelviureteric dilatation) in ureteral obstruction, it may not be possible to distinguish between these potential causes using gray-scale US alone. In other words, there may be non-obstructive dilatations, while collective system dilatation may not be observable despite the presence of obstruction. Moreover, in an acute context, obstruction may persist for several hours prior to collecting system dilatation. A number of teams in the early 1990s hypothesized that urinary obstruction pathophysiology could be reliably revealed by changes in arterial Doppler spectra (Platt et al., 1989a; 1989b; Platt, 1992; Rodgers et al., 1992). This was the result of exhaustive animal studies demonstrating unique biphasic hemodynamic response to complete ureteral obstruction.

5.2.1.1 Acute obstruction

Immediately after obstruction, renal blood flow increases in response to the elevation in ureteric pressure. This generally lasts less than 1.5–2 h. It is thought to be the result of preglomerular vasodilatation. This period of likely prostaglandin-mediated vasodilatation, lasting less than 2 h, occurs immediately after obstruction. The following 2–4 h sees a gradual fall in renal blood flow with continued elevation of pelvic and ureteric pressures, which are probably the result of postglomerular vasoconstriction. Kim et al. (1997) used unilateral lamb model an acutely obstructed and reported 29% decrease in total blood flow in the obstructed side, compared to an increase in total blood flow in the unobstructed kidney. Karaguzel et al. (2011) obtained similar findings using power Doppler in a study of partial unilateral ureteral obstruction in rabbits (Fig. 4.). This implies that resistance is increased on the obstructed side and reduced on the unobstructed side and that contralateral obstruction on the unobstructed kidney produces a notable effect. Renal blood flow thus declines, while renal vascular resistance increases. Initial research suggested that this vasoconstriction response was to a large extent a mechanical one, the result of increases in collecting system pressures. However, more recent studies suggest that complex interactions between several regulatory pathways (renin–angiotensin, kallikrein–kinin, and prostaglandin–thromboxane) are in fact responsible for intense, postobstructive renal vasoconstriction. Whatever the mediation involved, this vasoconstriction response appeared ideal for by changes in the RI. Researchers from University of Michigan obtained RIs from 21 hydronephrotic kidneys prior to nephrostomy. The mean RI levels in 14 kidneys with confirmed obstruction (0.77 ± 0.04) were higher compared to those from seven kidneys with non-obstructive pelvicaliectasis (0.64 ± 0.04). Additionally, intrarenal RI values returned to normal post-nephrostomy (Platt et al., 1989a). A subsequent larger study involving 229 kidneys largely corroborated these results. That study employed a discriminatory RI threshold of 0.70; sensitivity and specificity of the Doppler diagnosis of obstruction were determined as 92 and 88%, respectively (Platt et al., 1989b).

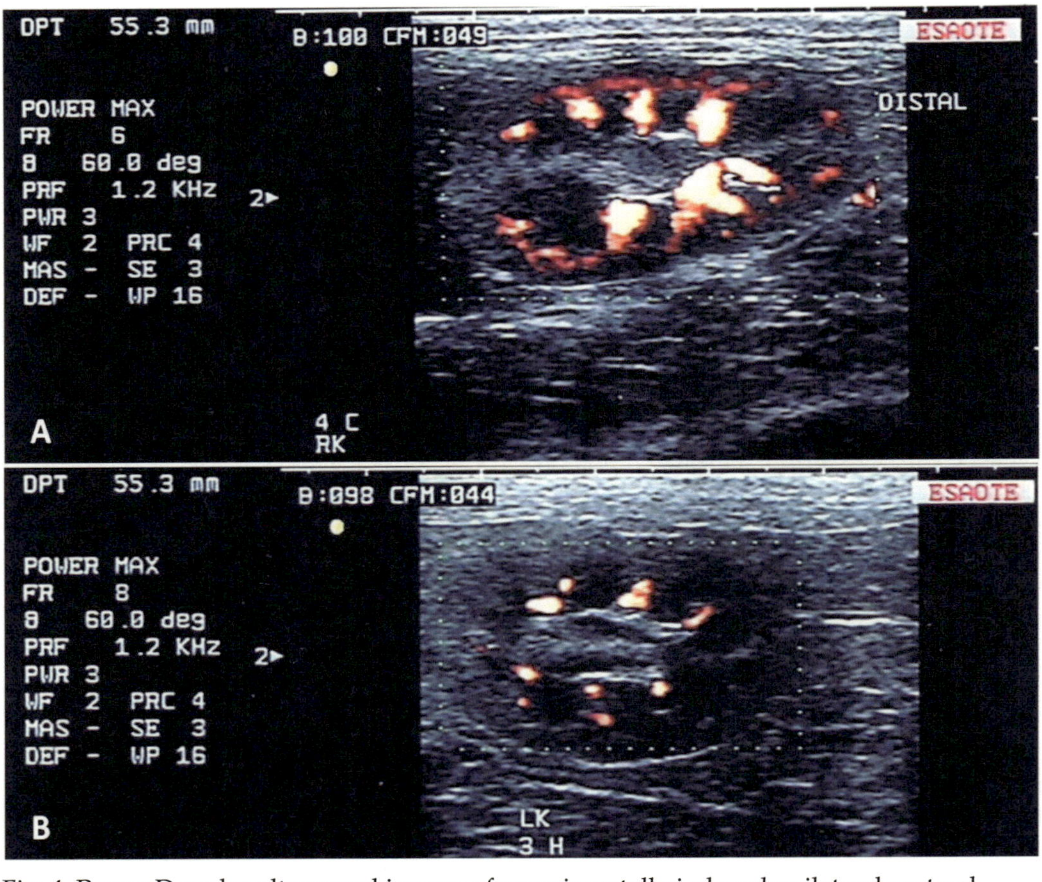

Fig. 4. Power Doppler ultrasound images of experimentally induced unilateral ureteral obstruction in a rabbit. Colorization in the non-obstructed right kidney (A) is clear, whereas in colorization of the interlobar vessels decreased and cortical colorization is absent in the obstructed left kidney (B) at 3 hr post-obstruction.

5.2.1.2 Ureteral obstruction severely dilating the collecting system

Severe hydronephrotic kidney was shown to not exhibit any elevation in intrarenal RI, despite the presence of what the authors regarded as obvious urinary obstruction (Platt et al., 1989b). The lack of response might have been due to a marked decrease in absolute blood flow in chronic high-grade obstruction, decreased filtration pressure produced by a renal cortex functioning at a minimal level or elevated compliance in a capacious dilated collecting system (Ulrich et al., 1995).

5.2.2 Partial ureteral obstruction

A number of reports (Brkljacic et al., 1994; Opdenakker et al., 1998; Rodgers et al., 1992; Shokeir & Abdulmaaboud, 2001) have encourage various institutions to include RI analysis in the sonographic evaluation of collecting system dilatation. However, anecdotal reports, follow-up clinical trials, and animal studies have all had a negative effect on the clinical impact of Doppler US (Chen et al., 1993; Cole et al., 1997; Coley et al., 1995; Deyoe et al., 1995; Rawashdeh et al., 2001; Tublin et al., 1994). Doppler US was found to be of especially limited use in the evaluation of partial ureteral obstruction. Chen et al. (1993), for example, reported a sensitivity of Doppler US for the diagnosis of obstruction of only 52%. Although the results of the examination were often positive with high-grade obstruction, most patients with partial obstruction had normal RIs. Doppler US's failure to reliably detect low-grade obstruction was confirmed later in pig and rabbit models (Cole et al., 1997; Coley et al., 1995; Kaya et al., 2010).

5.2.3 Comparison with the contralateral kidney without diuresis in obstuctive uropathy

The accuracy of the discriminatory value of RI (0.70) can be improved by evaluating the contralateral kidney. This is particularly the case in acute obstruction in which RI may still be below the limit of 0.70. A difference of ≥0.10 between the obstructed and the contralateral kidney further suggests the accuracy of the diagnosis (Platt et al., 1991a). Sensitivity rose from 57 to 71% in acute obstruction with comparison of RI in the two kidneys in one study (Rodgers et al., 1992). The obstructed to normal kidney RI ratio can also be helpful. Ulrich et al. (1995) cited a ration of 1.15 as a diagnostic criterion of acute obstruction. Keller et al. (1989) showed that with the RI ratio of ≥1.11, the sensitivity for determining obstruction was 77%, while the specificity for excluding obstruction was 81%, in a study involving 48 patients with unilateral obstruction and 34 healthy controls. Comparison with the contralateral kidney is not naturally used an option in patients with bilateral renal obstruction or with only one kidney (Shokeir et al., 1997a).

5.2.4 Diuresis in obstuctive uropathy (diuretic Doppler US)

A number of researchers have shown that it is possible to enhance the sensitivity of Doppler US for the detection of partial obstruction by performing the evaluation after forced diuresis (diuretic Doppler US) (Akata et al., 1999; Lee et al., 2001; Ordorica et al., 1993). Experimental research has provided a theoretical basis for the use of diuretic Doppler US in the evaluation of obstructive uropathy. An increase of RI of ≥15% after furosemide injection is regarded as a diagnostic criterion of obstruction (Ordorica et al., 1993). Infusion of normal saline and administration of furosemide have been shown to significantly enhance the sensitivity, specificity and general accuracy of the use of RI in the diagnosis of obstructed kidneys in children (Shokeir et al., 1996). Following induction of complete left-side ureteral obstruction, left intrarenal RI increased significantly over the course of five consecutive days. Mannitol has reduced intrarenal RI in the non-obstructed contralateral kidneys (Choi et al., 2003). The RI difference and ratio obtained in unilateral cases by comparison with the non-obstructive kidney further reinforces the diagnosis of obstructive uropathy. Fluid and diuretic procedures raise intrarenal RI values in the obstructed kidney. In this way, the further increase in RI difference and ratio that result are renal hemodynamic parameters that can be used in the diagnosis of unilateral ureteral obstruction. (Kaya et al., 2010)

Palmer et al. (1991) investigated Doppler US in children before and after the administration of intravenous furosemide. They demonstrated that this leads to an increase in RI above baseline in obstructed kidneys, but that it has no significant impact on RI compared to baseline in normal and non-obstructed pyelocliectasic kidneys. Bude et al. (1994) showed that infusion of normal saline and administration of furosemide reduced intrarenal RI of non-obstructed renal units to a significant extent compared with baseline values. In the wake of such positive, further series indicated the potential of Doppler US to differentiate renal transplant obstructive and non-obstructive pelvicaliectasis (Platt et al., 1991c) and to determine ureteral stent patency (Platt et al., 1993).

5.2.5 Changes in renal resistive index following relief of obstruction

Platt et al. (1989a) reported that 2–9 days after the relief of obstruction RI decreased in nine out of 10 adult patients. Ordorica et al. (1993) showed that RI decreased to <0.75 in all nine kidneys evaluated 3 months after operation. Shokeir et al. (1997b) also confirmed that RI reversed after relief of mild and severe degrees of obstruction in an experimental model. An experimental study in dogs reported that elevated intrarenal RI value in complete bilateral ureteral obstruction was not affected by peritoneal dialysis, but this high level again decreased with relief of the obstruction (Kirmizigul et al., 2007). On the other hand, Chen et al. (1993) reported that RI remained elevated in two out of five adult patients after the release of obstruction. Future studies might usefully determine those factors interfering with the reversal of RI after the relief of obstruction, such as the age of the patient, the type and duration of obstruction, and the extent of vascular and parenchymal damage.

5.2.6 The effect of certain drugs on renal resistive index in obstuctive uropathy

Patients who present with renal colic with are often administered with non-steroidal anti-inflammatory drugs (NSAIDs) for pain relief prior to undergoing a comprehensive diagnostic evaluation. NSAIDs reduce prostaglandin synthesis, and are therefore involved in hemodynamic changes within the kidney, with resultant changes in the renovascular resistance. This can thus impact on intrarenal RI. These drugs can reverse both the early vasodilatation and later vasoconstriction that accompany acute renal obstruction and hence lower renal blood flow, renal vascular resistance and glomerular filtration rate. Low urine production causes lower intraluminal pressure, one of the major causes of renal obstruction (Kmetec at al., 2002). Shokeir et al. (1999) reported that NSAIDs significantly decreased the RI of acutely obstructed kidneys, but did not affect RI in normal contralateral kidneys. However, although their patients were administered ketoprofen, mean RI levels for the obstructed kidneys remained above the discriminatory threshold (>0.70) during the first 71 h of obstruction (Kmetec et al., 2002). The mean RI on the obstructed side was only slightly below the threshold in kidneys obstructed for > 72 h, though the difference between the kidneys was significant. On the basis of their findings, the measurement of RI is a trustworthy diagnostic method for detecting acute renal obstruction.

In a study on rabbits, Ayyıldız et al. (2009) stated that tadalafil had a low effect on intrarenal RI and PI in partial ureteral obstruction. They suggested that their findings might lead to this drug being used to minimize the negative effects of obstruction in clinical practice. Another study suggested that ginkgo glycosides may protect and restore renal perfusion in partial unilateral ureteral obstructions, as shown by a decrease in RI and the enhanced colorization obtained with power Doppler US in the obstructed kidney. That study further suggested that ginkgo glycosides might also be employed to minimize renal parenchymal damage and maintain kidney function (Karaguzel et al., 2011).

5.2.7 Changes in venous impedance caused by obstuctive uropathy

The intrarenal venous impedance index determined by the use of Doppler US is associated with compliance in the vein and can assist in assessing renal parenchymal compliance (Karabulut et al., 2003). Researchers have observed a dampening of the hepatic vein signal in cases of acute and chronic liver disease, and have ascribed this to reduced hepatic compliance (Bolondi et al., 1991). It has been suggested that, because of the resulting changes in compliance, disease in the liver can be identified by measuring the pulsatility of the venous signal in the hepatic veins. Compliance of the liver tissue is reflected by the pulsatility of the hepatic venous signal since the majority of pathologies expand the liver parenchyma within its confining capsule. This, in turn, reduces compliance and leads to dampening of the hepatic venous signal (Britton et al., 1992). It is believed that there is an equivalent phenomenon in the kidney. It has been suggested that the increased pressure causing a decrease in renal parenchymal compliance in acute renal obstructions may also alter Doppler signals obtained from the intrarenal veins (Bateman & Cuganesen, 2002; Karabulut et al., 2003). Right-sided atrial pressure changes result in a triphasic waveform. In this situation, the atrial and sometimes the ventricular venous pulse components produce a reversed flow in the inferior vena cava (Appleton et al., 1987). The reversal of flow at the end of diastole (from atrial contraction) progresses into the renal vessels. The arterial data also show a high flow of blood into the kidney throughout diastole and that enlargement of the veins (compliance) has to compensate for a temporary decrease in outflow. If the veins are made non-compliant due to raised interstitial pressure, this end diastolic flow reduction declines. Similarly, venous pulsatility rises if compliance is increased (Bateman and Cuganesen 2002). Once peak venous flow signal (A) and least flow signal (B) (Fig. 3) have been measured venous impedance index (A-B/A) is calculated (Bateman and Cuganesen 2002, Karabulut et al. 2003). The venous impedance indices (0.44 ± 0.06 for the right kidney, 0.41 ± 0.07 for the left kidney) determined for the normal kidney by Karabulut et al. (2003) were compatible with those from an earlier study by Bateman and Cuganesen (2002), who reported mean impedance indices of 0.45 ± 0.18 for the right kidney and 0.43 ± 0.19 for the left kidney. Bateman & Cuganesan (2002) further reported venous impedance indices of 0.38 ± 0.25 for the obstructed side and 0.80 ± 0.25 for the unobstructed side. The peak venous flow signal in the obstructed kidney was 69% higher than the flow in the unobstructed kidney and 86% higher than the signal in the control group. They suggested that renal obstruction produces a greater change in venous flow than arterial flow, and concluded that a comparison between venous flow levels in the obstructed and unobstructed kidneys might result in enhanced diagnostic accuracy.

6. Doppler ultrasonographic examination of renal allograft

Kidney transplant is the treatment of choice for patients with end-stage renal disease. These patients are susceptible to complications with the potential to threaten the transplant kidney, especially immediately after transplant. The main allograft complications are vascular pathology (renal artery stenosis or occlusion, renal vein thrombosis, arteriovenous fistulas and pseudoaneurism), collecting system pathology and medical allograft dysfunctions (rejection, acute tubular necrosis, cyclosporine toxicity, and infection). These complications are routinely differentiated using renal biopsy, though the procedure is invasive and poses inherent morbidity risks. The usefulness of renal Doppler US as a noninvasive technique in the evaluation of these complications has been established. The RI value is a sensitive index in predicting renal allograft dysfunction.

6.1 Vascular system pathologies in renal transplantation

6.1.1 Renal artery stenosis or occlusion

Doppler US findings for transplant kidney in the main renal artery stenosis or occlusions are to a great extent similar to those for the native kidney. However, transplant kidneys possess a number of advantages making Doppler ultrasonographic diagnosis more definitive. The first of these is that the transplant kidney and its arterial structures can be more clearly visualized sonographically. The absence from the transplant kidney of collateral arterial structures present in the native kidney and a knowledge of the artery number and localizations of anastomoses means that the main renal arteries can be distinguished and evaluated easily and reliably. The presence of intrarenal Doppler findings such as late elevation of systolic peak, low flow velocity, pulsus tardus *et* parvus, a decrease in flow velocity, low RI (<0.50) and PI values, decreased acceleration (<3 m/s^2), and increased acceleration time (>70 m/s) will suggest renal artery pathologies (Bude and Rubin 1995; Handa et al.1986). Following the determination of these Doppler findings the renal artery has to be evaluated with Doppler US. Renal artery systolic velocity needs to be correlated with the systolic velocity of the iliac artery in the proximal direction (renoiliac ratio) as a renal artery stenosis finding. A ratio greater than 2 has been proposed as a diagnostic criterion in renal artery stenosis (Gottlieb et al., 1995; McGee et al., 1990). Helenon et al. (1994) reported that although Doppler ultrasonographic diagnosis had a more limited success rate in stenosis in the segmental branches it had an almost 100% diagnostic success rate in renal artery stenosis.

6.1.2 Renal vein thrombosis

Renal vein thrombosis, one of the early complications of the transplant kidney, can lead to loss of the transplant kidney if diagnosis is delayed. Because the transplant kidney has advantages over the native kidney with regard to sonographic imaging, renal Doppler US is quite successful in revealing this pathology. In contrast to the native kidney, because the transplant kidney has no collateral vascular structures and possibility of drainage, renal vein and intrarenal Doppler US findings are more dramatic (Helenon et al., 1995). If the diastolic flow component is below the baseline (reversed flow form), this spectral image is a non-specific finding in acute rejection and acute tubular necrosis (Schwerk et al., 1994). Renal vein thrombosis may be present when diastolic flow is reversed and no renal venous flow is detected (Dodd et al., 1991b).

6.1.3 Arteriovenous fistulas and pseudoaneurisms

Transplant kidneys are frequently subjected to biopsy during or after transplantation. Arteriovenous fistulas and pseudoaneurisms that generally arise in association with renal biopsy are evaluated in terms of the criteria used in Doppler ultrasonographic diagnosis of arteriovenous fistulas and pseudoaneurisms in the native kidney. For example, focal high velocity, low-impedance intrarenal arterial flow might suggest an arteriovenous fistula. At the same time, because of the imaging advantages attendant upon the transplant kidney diagnosis can easily be established.

6.2 Collecting system pathologies in renal transplantation

Since the transplant kidney is removed together with the ureters during surgery and anastomosed to the recipient bladder at a different level (ureteroneocystostomy), mild pelvicaliectasis and ureter dilatation may be determined in the anastomosis region in the early postoperative period. Another possible cause of these ultrasonographic findings is that the kidney and ureters are significantly denerved and the collective system loses natural tonus. In contrast, obstructive pathologies may cause significant pelvicaliectasis and/or ureter dilatation. One finding in respect of obstructive transplant kidney pathologies that must not be underestimated is the possibility of renal colic in the denerved kidneys. Obstruction in these kidneys, where urine output is at the threshold limit, prevents the collecting system being dilated with urine as a cause of a sudden drop in output. Repeated rejection attacks cause the walls of the collecting system and ureter to thicken and lose elasticity. Therefore, collecting system dilatation may not be observed in transplant kidneys with obstructive pathology (Bude & Rubin, 1995). In contrast to these ultrasound findings in obstruction, an abnormal rise may be seen in Doppler indices during the early postoperative period. However, the rise in these indices may also be seen in medical pathologies (*e.g.*, rejection) (Platt et al., 1991c).

6.3 Medical allograft dysfunctions

These patients must be properly monitored and screened in the early postoperative period for management of early onset renal complications and dysfunctions. It is important to begin a work-up to establish the precise nature of the problem and determine the optimal management as soon as possible. The use of a non-invasive technique capable of accurately establishing and identifying the causes of renal transplant dysfunction is also important. While renal biopsy is the standard means of distinguishing between these complications, it is nevertheless invasive and involves inherent risks of morbidity. Conventional US is able to determine anatomical changes in the allograft (hydronephrosis, hematoma and urinoma, for instance), but it is less successful in evaluating functional abnormalities, such as acute tubular necrosis, acute rejection, and drug toxicity (Radmehr et al., 2008). Initial enthusiasm gradually gave way to skepticism over a number of articles investigating the role of Doppler US in transplant dysfunction analysis (Allen et al., 1998; Buckly et al., 1987; Choi et al., 1998; Rifkin et al., 1987; Rigsby et al., 1987; Trillaud et al. 1998).

6.3.1 Rejection

Acute rejection represents the most common need for special attention. Elevated RI used to be regarded as specific for rejection (Allen et al., 1998; Buckly et al., 1987; Rifkin et al., 1987).

A number of studies have subsequently revealed the lack of specificity inherent in an elevated RI (Choi et al., 1998; Trillaud et al., 1998). Perrella et al. (1990), for example, reported that sensitivity and specificity of Doppler US for the diagnosis of rejection was 43 and 67%, respectively, with a threshold RI of 0.90. The complex and heterogeneous nature of rejection physiopathology may be regarded as responsible for this discrepancy. One study showed that Doppler indices may be initially normal, and even low, at the beginning of the pathology in mild-moderate intensity acute rejection (Ponziak et al., 1992). Because of these discouraging results, most physicians regard an elevated RI as a nonspecific marker of transplant dysfunction. It has been maintained that renal vascular resistance is not static, in acute rejection, but exhibits a dynamic picture depending on such variables as the immunosuppressive drugs used and the degree of rejection. Accordingly, reports have stated that values from Doppler examinations obtained at different times in cases of acute rejection may be of greater use in diagnosis (Hollenbeck, 1994; Mizrahi et al., 1993). Although RI analysis is not helpful in differentiating the typical causes of transplant dysfunction (acute tubular necrosis, rejection, and immunosuppression toxicity), it is still useful for identifying vascular complications associated with transplantation.

6.3.2 Acute tubular necrosis

Acute tubular necrosis is common in transplant kidneys from cadaver donors. It is a primary allograft dysfunction. Diuresis either never develops, or else is soon halted. Although these preliminary clinical findings are supported by elevated renal Doppler indices, no typical finding has been described for acute tubular necrosis in practice (Lee & Newstead, 1993; Taylor &Marks, 1990).

6.3.3 Other allograft complications

In the late postoperative period, a series of allograft dysfunctions, such as chronic rejection, cyclosporine toxicity and glomerulonephritis, developing in the allograft kidney present a similar pathological picture. Success levels in studies regarding definitive diagnosis and differentiation of these pathologies with Doppler US are not at all high (Pelling & Dubbins, 1992; Taylor & Marks, 1990).

7. Conclusion

As a noninvasive technique, renal Doppler US allows evaluation of renal hemodynamics, which helps to diagnose and monitor renal pathologies. Based on earlier clinical and experimental studies, Doppler ultrasonographic parameters have today been identified and defined as diagnostic indices for determining renal hemodynamic changes in response to renal vascular pathologies. When diuretic procedures together with RI difference and ratio are used in unilateral ureteral obstruction, renal Doppler US may be enough to make an accurate diagnosis. However, this technique should be combined with other radiological methods in patients with bilateral renal obstruction. Moreover, in the evaluation of both native and transplant kidneys, renal Doppler US has assumed the important function of concentrating suspicions on renal medical pathologies by successfully excluding vascular and obstructive pathologies.

8. References

Aikimbaev KS, Canataroglu A, Ozbek S & Usal A. (2001). Renal Vascular Resistance in Progressive Systemic Sclerosis: Evaluation with Duplex Doppler Ultrasound. Angiology 52: 697-701.

Akata D, Haliloglu M, Caglar M, Tekgul S, Ozmen MN & Akhan O. (1999). Renal Diuretic Duplex Doppler Sonography in Childhood Hydronephrosis. Acta Radiol 40:203-206.

Allen K, Jorkasky D, Arger P, Velchik MG, Grumbach K, Coleman BG, Mintz MC, Betsch SE & Perloff LJ. (1988). Renal Allografts: Prospective Analysis of Doppler Sonography. Radiology 169:371-376.

Alterini B, Mori F, Terzani E, Raineri M, Zuppiroli A, De Saint Pierre G, Favilli S, D'Agata A & Fazzini G. (1996). Renal Resistive Index and Left Ventricular Hypertrophy in Essential Hypertension: A Close Link. Ann Ital Med Int 11:107-113.

Andriani G, Persico A, Tursini S, Ballone E, Cirotti D & Lelli Chiesa P. (2001). The Renal Resistive Index from the Last 3 Months of Pregnancy to 6 Months Old. BJU Int 87:562-564.

Appleton CP, Hatle LK & Popp RL. (1987). Superior Vena Cava and Hepatic Vein Doppler Echocardiography in Healthy Adults. J Am Coll Cardiol 10:1032-1039.

Ayyildiz A, Kaya M, Karaguzel E, Bumin A, Akgul T, Alkan Z & Germiyanoglu C.(2009). Effect of Tadanafil on Renal Resistivity and Pulsatility Index in Partial Ureteral Obstruction. Urol Inter 83:75-79.

Avasthi PS, Voyles WF & Greene JH. (1984). Noninvasive Diagnosis of Renal Artery Stenosis by Echo-Doppler Velocimetry. Kidney 25:824-829.

Bateman GA & Cuganesan R. (2002). Renal Vein Doppler Sonography of Obstructive Uropathy. AJR 178:921-925.

Bolondi L, Bassi SL, Gaiani S, Zironi G, Benzi G, Santi V & Barbara L. (1991). Liver Cirrhosis: Changes of Doppler Waveform of Hepatic Veins. Radiology 178:513-516.

Britton PD, Lomas DJ, Coulden RA & Revell S. (1992). The Role of Hepatic Vein Doppler in Diagnosing Acute Rejection Following Paediatric Liver Transplantion. Clin Radiol 45:228-232.

Brkljacic B, Drinkovic I, Sabjar-Matovianovic M, Soldo D, Morovic-Vergles J,Vidjak V & Hebrang A. (1994). Intrarenal Duplex Doppler Sonographic Evaluation of Unilateral Native Kidney Obstruction. J Ultrasound Med 13:197-204.

Buckley A, Cooperberg P, Reeve C & Magil AB. (1987). The Distinction between Acute Renal Transplant Rejection and Cyclosporine Nephrotoxicity: Value of Duplex Sonography. AJR 149:521-525.

Bude RO, DiPietro MA, Platt JF, Rubin JM, Miesowicz S & Lundquist C. (1992). Age Dependency of the Renal Resistive Index in Healthy Children. Radiology 184:469-73.

Bude RO, DiPietro MA & Platt JF. (1994). Effect of Furosemide and Intravenous Normal Saline Load upon the Renal Resistive Index in Nonobstructed Kidneys in Children. J Urol 151:438-441.

Bude RO & Rubin JM. (1995). Detection of Renal Artery Stenosis with Doppler Sonography: It is More Complicated Than Orginally Thought. Radiology 196:612-613.

Bude RO & Rubin JM. (1999). Relationship between the Resistive Index and Vascular Compliance and Resistance. Radiology 211:411-417.

Carvalho CF & Chammas MC. (2011). Normal Doppler Velocimetry of Renal Vasculature in Persian Cats. J Feline Med Surg 13:399-404.

Chang YJ, Chan IP, Cheng FP, Wang WS, Liu CP & Lin SL. (2010). Relationship between Age, Plasma Renin Activity, and Renal Resistive Index in Dogs. Vet Radiol Ultrasound. 51:335-337.

Chen P, Maklad N & Redwine M. (1998). Color and Power Doppler Imaging of the Kidneys. World J UrolP 16: 41-45.

Chen J, Pu Y, Liu S & Chin TY. (1993). Renal Hemodynamics in Patients with Obstructive Uropathy Evaluated by Duplex Doppler Sonography. J Urol 150:18-21.

Choi CS, Lee S & Kim JS. (1998). Usefulness of the Resistive Index for the Evaluation of Transplanted Kidneys. Transplant Proc 30:3074-3075

Choi H, Won S, Chung W, Lee K, Chang D, Lee H, Eom K, Lee Y & Yoon J. (2003). Effect of Intravenous Mannitol upon the Resistive Index in Complete Unilateral Renal Obstruction in Dogs. J Vet Intern Med 17:158-162.

Chu Y, Liu H, Xing P, Lou G & Wu C. (2011). The Morhology and Haemodynamics of The Rabbit Renal Artery: Evaluation by Conventional and Contrast-Enhanced US. Lab Anim 45:204-208.

Claudon M, Barnewolt CE, Taylor GA, Dunning PS, Boget R & Badawy AB. (1999). Renal Blood Flow in Pigs: Changes Depicted with Contrast-Enhanced Harmonic US Imaging during Acute Urinary Obstruction. Radiology 212:725-731.

Claudon M, Plouin PF, Baxter GM, Rohban T & Devos DM. (2000). Renal Arteries in Patients at Risk of Renal Arterial Stenosis: Multicenter Evaluation of the Echo-Enhancer SH U 508A at Color and Spectral Doppler US. Levovist Renal Artery Stenosis Study Group. Radiology 214:739-746.

Cole T, Brock J & Pope J. (1997). Evaluation of Renal Resistive Index, Maximum Velocity, and Mean Arterial Flow Velocity in a Hydronephrotic Partially Obstructed Pig Model. Invest Radiol 32:154-160.

Coley B, Arellano R, Talner L, Baker KG, Peterson T & Mattrey RF. (1995). Renal Resistive Index in Experimental Partial and Complete Ureteral Obstruction. Acad Radiol 2:373-378.

Daley CA, Finn-Bodner ST & Lenz SD. (1994). Contrast-induced Renal Failure Documented by Color-Doppler imaging in a Dog. J Am Anim Hosp Assoc 30: 33-37

Derchi LE, Martinoli C & Saffioti S. (1994). Ultrasonographic Imaging and Doppler Analysis of Renal Changes in Non-Insuline Dependent Diabetes Mellitus. Acad Radiol. 1: 100-107.

Deyoe L, Cronan J, Breslaw B & Ridlen MS. (1995). New Techniques of Ultrasound and Color Doppler in the Prospective Evaluation of Acute Renal Obstruction: Do They Replace the Intravenous Urogram? Abdom Imaging 20:58-63.

Dodd GD, Kaufman PN & Bracken RB. (1991a). Renal Arterial Duplex Doppler Ultrasound in Dogs with Urinary Obstruction. J Urol 145: 644-646.

Dodd G, Tublin M, Shah A & Zajko AB. (1991b). Imaging of Vascular Complications Associated with Renal Transplants. AJR 157:449-459.

Edwards D & Beggs I. (1987). Renal Vascular Disease: Miscellaneous Lessions, In Sutton D (Ed.) Atextbook of Radiology and Imaging. Edinburg, Scotland, Churchill Livingstone. p 1169.

Fiselier T, Derkx F, Monnens L, Van Munster P, Peer P & Schalekamp M. (1984). The Basal Levels of Active and Inactive Plasma Renin Concentration in İnfancy and Childhood. Clin Sci 67:383-387.

Frauchiger B, Nussbaumer P, Hugentobler M & Staub D. (2000). Duplex Sonographic Registration of Age and Diabetes-Related Loss of Renal Vasodilatory Response to Nitroglycerine. Nephrol Dial Transplant 15:827-832.

Gonul R, Koenhemsi L, Bayrakal A, Bahceci T, Erman M & Uysal A. (2011). Renal-Pulsed Wave Doppler Ultrasonographic Findings of Normal Turkish Angora Cats. Pak Vet J 31:369-370.

Gottlieb RH, Lieberman JL, Pabico RC & Waldman DL. (1995). Diagnosis of Renal Artery Stenosis in Transplanted Kidney: Value of Doppler Waveform Analysis of the Intrarenal Arteries. AJR 165:1441-1446.

Handa N, Fukunaga R, Uehara A, Etani H, Yoneda S, Kimura K & Kamada T. (1986). Echo-Doppler Velocimeter in the Diagnosis of Hypertensive Patient: The Renal Artery Doppler Technique. Ultrasound Med Biol. 12:945-952.

Helenon O, Correas JM, Melki PH, Thervet E, Churetien Y & Moreau JF. (1994). Value of Color Doppler US in the Diagnosis Renal Transplant artery stenosis. Ultrasound Med Biol 20:83-89.

Helenon O, Rody FE & Correas JM. (1995). Color Doppler US of Renovascular Disease in Native Kidneys. Radiographics 15:833-854.

Hollenbeck M. (1994). New Diagnostic Techniques in Clinic Nephrology. Colour Coded Duplex Sonography for Evaluation of Renal Transplants-tool Fort He Nephrologist? Nephrol Dial Transplant. 9:1822-1828.

House MK, Dowling RJ, King PM, Bourke JL & Gibson RN. (1999). Contrast-enhanced Doppler Ultrasound for Renal Artery Stenosis. Australas Radiol 43:206-209.

Kaya M, Pekcan Z, Sen Y, Boztok B, Senel OO & Bumin A. (2011). Effects of Short-Acting Anaesthetics on Haemodynamic Function as Determined by Doppler US in Rabbits. Kafkas Univ Vet Fak Derg 17:713-719.

Kaya M, Bumin A, Sen Y & Alkan Z. (2010). Comparison of Excretory Urography, US-Guided Percutaneous Antegrade Pyelography, and Renal Doppler US in Rabbits with Unilateral Partial Ureteral Obstruction: An Experimental Study. Kafkas Univ Vet Fak Derg 16:735-741.

Karabulut N, Yagcı AB & Karabulut A. (2003). Renal Vein Doppler Ultrasound of Maternal Kidney in Normal Second and Third Trimester Pregnancy. British J Radiol 76:444-447.

Karaguzel E, Kaya M, Bumin A & Ayyildiz A. (2011). *Ginko Biloba* extract maintains renal perfusion in partial unilateral ureteral obstructions. Bull Vet Inst Pullawy 55: 273-279.

Keller MS, Garcia CJ, Korsvik H, Weiss RM & Rosenfield NS. (1991). Resistive Index Ratios in the US Differantiation of Unilateral Obstructive vs Non-obstructive Hydronephrosis in Children. Ped Radiol 21:462-466.

Keogan M, Kliewer M, Hertzberg B, DeLong DM, Tupler RH & Carroll BA. (1996a). Renal resistive indexes: variability in Doppler US measurement in a healthy population. Radiology 199:165-169.

Keogan M, Hertzberg B, Kliewer M, DeLong DM, Paulson EK & Carrol BA. (1996b). Doppler Sonography in the diagnosis of antepartum pyelonephritis: Value of Intrarenal Resistive Index Measurents. J Ultrasound Med 15:13-17.

Kier R, Taylor KJW, Feyock AL & Ramos IM. (1990). Renal Masses: Characterization with Doppler US. Radiology 176:703-707.

Kim S, Kim W, Choi B & Kim CW. (1992). Duplex Sonography of the Native Kidney: Resistive Index vs Serum Creatinine. Clin Radiol 45:85-87.

Kim KM, Bogaert GA, Nguyen HT, Borirakchanyavat S & Kogan BA. (1997). Hemodynamic Changes after Complete Unilateral Ureteral Obstruction in the Young Lamb. J Urol 158:1090-1093.

Kirmizigul AH, Kaya M, Bumin A & Kalınbacak A. (2007). Evaluation of Resistive Index Parameter in Peritoneal Dialysis in Dogs with Experimental Bilateral Proximal Ureteral Obstruction. Kafkas Üniv Vet Fak Derg 13:33-38.

Kmetec A, Babnik DP & Ponikvar JB. (2002). Time-dependent Changes of Resistive Index in Acute Renal Obstruction During Nonsteroidal Drug Administration. BJU Intern 89:847-850.

Krumme B, Blum U, Schwertfeger E, Flügel P, Höllstin F, Schollmeyer P & Rump LC. (1996). Diagnosis of Renovascular Disease by Intra- and Extrarenal Doppler Scanning. Kidney Int 50:1288-1292.

Kuzmic AC, Brkljacic B, Ivankovic D & Galesic K. (2000). Doppler Sonographic Renal Resistance Index in Healthy Children. Eur Radiol 10:1644-8.

Lee SH & Newstead CG. (1993). Case Repot: Sonographic Detection in Renal Transplant Cortical Calcification. Clin Radiol 47:207-208.

Lee HJ, Cho JY & Kim SH. (2001). Resistive index in rabbits with experimentally induced hydronephrosis: effect of furosemide. Acad Radiol 8:987-992

Marzano MA, Pompili M & Rapaccini GL. (1998). Early Renal Involvement in Diabetes Mellitus: Comparison of Renal Doppler US and Radioisotope Evaluation of Glomerular Hyperfiltration. Radiology 209:813-817.

McGee GS, Peterson-Kennedy L, Astleford P & Yao JST. (1990). Duplex Assesment of the Renal Transplant. Surg Clin N Am 70: 133-141.

Melany ML, Grant EG, Duerinckx AJ, Watts TM & Levine BS. (1997). Ability of a Phase Shift US Contrast Agent to Improve Imaging of the Main Renal Arteries. Radiology 205: 147-152.

Miralles M, Cairols M, Cotillas J, Giménez A & Santiso A. (1996). Value of Doppler Parameters in the Diagnosis of Renal Artery Stenosis. J Vasc Surg 23:428-35.

Missouris CG, Allen CM, Balen FG, Buckenham T, Lees WR & MacGregor GA. (1996). Non-invasive screening for Renal Artery Stenosis with Ultrasound Contrast Enhancement. J Hypertens 14: 519-524.

Mitchell SK, Toal RL, Daniel GB & Rohrbach BW. (1998). Evaluation of renal hemodynamics in awake and isofluorane-anesthetized cats with pulsedwave Doppler and quantitative renal scintigraphy. Vet Radiol Ultrasound 39:451-458.

Mizrahi S, Hussey JL & Hayes DH. (1993). Protocol Doppler Color Flow Imaging Immidiately after Kidney Transplantation. South Med J 86: 1126-1128.

Morrow Kl, Salman MD, Lappin MR & Wrigley R. (1996). Comparison of the Resistive Index to Clinical Parameters in Dogs with Renal Disease. Vet Radiol Ultrasound 37:193-199.

Mostbeck GH Gossinger HD, Mallek R, Siostrzonek P, Schneider B & Tscholakoff D. (1990). Effect of Heart Rate on Doppler Measurments of Resistive Index in Renal Arteries. Radiology 175:511-513.

Murat A, Akarsu S, Ozdemir H, Yildirim H & Kalender O. (2005). Renal Resistive Index in Healthy Children. Eur J Radiol 53:67-71.

Murphy ME & Tublin ME. (2000). Understanding the Doppler RI: Impact of Renal Arterial Distensibility on the RI in a Hydronephrotic Ex-vivo Rabbit Kidney Model. J Ultrasound Med 19:303-314.

Norris C, Pfeiffer J, Rittgers S & Barnes RW. (1984). Noninvasive Evaluation of Renal Artery Stenosis and Renovascular Resistance: Experimental and Clinical Studies. J Vasc Surg 1:192-201

Novellas R, Espada Y & Gopegui RR. (2007). Doppler Ultrasonographic Estimation of Renal and Ocular Resistive and Pulsative Indices in Normal Dogs and Cats. Vet Radiol Ultrasound 48: 69-73.

Nyland TG, Fisher PE & Doverspike M. (1993) Diagnosis of Urinary Tract Obstruction in Dogs Using Duplex Doppler US. Vet Radiol Ultrasound 34:348-352.

Okten A, Dinc H, Kul M, Kaya G & Can G. (1999). Renal Duplex Doppler US as a Predictor of Preclinical Diabetic Nephropathy in Children. Acta Radiol 40:246-249.

Opdenakker L, Oyen R & Vervloessem I. (1998). Acute Obstruction of the Renal Collecting System: The Intrarenal Resistive Index is a Useful yet Time-dependent parameter for Diagnosis. Eur Radiol 8:1429-1432.

Ordorica R, Lindfors K & Palmer J. (1993). Diuretic Doppler Sonography following Successful Repair of Renal Obstruction in Children. J Urol 150:774-777.

Ozbek SS, Aytaç SK, Erden MI & Sanlıdilek U. (1993). Intrarenal Doppler Findings of Upstream Renal Artery Stenosis: A Preliminary Report. Ultrasound Med Biol 19: 3-12.

Ozbek SS, Memiş A, Killi R, Karaca E, Kabasakal C & Mir S. (1995). Image-directed and color Doppler US in the Diagnosis of Postbiopsy Arteriovenous Fistulas of Native kidneys. J Clin Ultrasound 23: 239-242.

Park IN, Lee HS, Kim JK, Nam SJ, Choi R, Oh KS, Son CH & Hyun C. (2008). Ultrasonographic Evaluation of Renal Dimension and Resistive Index in Clinically Healthy Korean Domestic Short-hair Cats. J Vet Sci 9: 415-419.

Patriquin H, O'Regan S, Robitaille P & Paltiel H. (1989). Hemolytic-uremic Syndrome: Intrarenal Arterial Doppler Patterns as a Useful Guide to Therapy. Radiology 172: 625-628.

Pelling M & Dubbins PA. (1992). Doppler and Color Doppler Imaging in Acute Transplant Failure. J Clin Ultrasound 20: 507-516.

Perrella R, Duerincky A & Tessler F. (1990). Evaluation of Renal Transplant Dysfunction by Duplex Doppler Sonography: a Prospective Study and Review of the Literature. Am J Kidney Dis 15:544-550.

Petersen LJ, Petersen JR, Ladefoged SD, Mehlsen J & Jensen HA. (1995). The Pulsatility Index and the Resistive Index in Renal Arteries in Patients with Hypertension and Chronic Renal Failure. Nephrol Dial Transplant 10: 2060-2064.

Platt J, Rubin J, Ellis J & DiPietro MA. (1989a). Duplex Doppler US of the Kidney; Differentiation of Obstructive from Nonobstructive Dilatation. Radiology 171:515-517.

Platt JF, Rubin JM & Ellis JH. (1989b). Distinction between Obstructive and Nonobstructive Pyelocaliectasis with Duplex Doppler Sonography. AJM 153:997-1000.

Platt J, Ellis J, Rubin J, DiPietro MA & Sedman AB. (1990). Intrarenal Arterial Doppler Sonography in Patients with Nonobstructive Renal Disease: Correlation of Resistive Index with Biopsy Findings. AJR 154:1223-1227.

Platt J, Ellis J & Rubin J. (1991a). Examination of Native Kidneys with Duplex Doppler Ultrasound. Semin Ultrasound CT MR 12:308-318

Platt J, Rubin J & Ellis J. (1991b). Acute Renal Failure: Possible Role of Duplex Doppler US in Distinction between Acute Prerenal Failure and Acute Tubular Necrosis. Radiology 179:419-423.

Platt J, Ellis J & Rubin J. (1991c). Renal Transplant Pyelocaliectasis: Role of Duplex Doppler US in Evaluation. Radiology 179:425-428

Platt J. (1992). Doppler evaluation of native kidney dysfunction: obstructive and nonobstructive disease. AJR 158:1035-1042.

Platt J, Marn C, Baliga P, Ellis JH, Rubin JM & Merion RM. (1992). Renal Dysfunction in Hepatic Disease: Early Identification with Renal Duplex Doppler US in Patients Who Undergo Liver Transplantation. Radiology 183:801-806.

Platt JF, Ellis JH & Rubin JM. (1993). Assessment of Internal Ureteral Stent Patency in Patients with Pyelocaliectasis: Value of Renal Duplex Sonography. AJR 161:87-90.

Platt JF, Rubin JM & Ellis JH. (1994a).Diabetic nephropathy: Evaluation with Renal Duplex Doppler US. Radiology 190: 343-346.

Platt JF, Ellis JH, Rubin JM, Merion RM & Lucey MR. (1994b). Renal Duplex Doppler US: A Noninvasive Predictor of Kidney Dysfunction and Hepatorenal Failure in Liver Disease. Hepatology 20:362-369.

Platt J, Rubin J & Ellis J. (1997). Lupus Nephritis: Predictive Value of Conventional and Doppler US and Comparison with Serologic and Biopsy Parameters. Radiology 203:82-86.

Pontremoki R, Viazzi F & Martinoli C. (1999). Increased Renal Resistive Index in Patients with Essential Hypertension: a Marker of Target Organ Damage. Nephrol Dial Transplant 14:360-365.

Pope JC, Hernanz-Schulman M, Showalter PR, Cole TC, Schrum FF, Szurkus D & Brock JW. (1996). The Value of Doopler Resistive Index and Peak Systolic Velocity in the Evaluation of Porcine Renal Obstruction. J Urol. 156:730-733.

Pozniak MA, Kelcz F & Stratta RJ. (1988). Extraneous Factors Affecting Resistive Index. Invest Radiol. 23: 899-901.

Ponziak MA, Kelcz F, D'Alessandro A, Oberley T & Stratta R. (1992). Sonography of Renal Transplants in Dogs: The Effect of Acute Tubular Necrosis. Cyclosporine Neprotoxicity, and Acute Rejection on Resistive Index and Renal Length. AJR 158:791-797.

Radmehr A, Jandaghi AB, Taheri APH & Shakiba M. (2008). Serial Resistive Index and Pulsatility Index for Diagnosing Renal Complications in the Early Posttransplant Phase: Improving Diagnostic Efficacy by Considering Maximum Values. Exp Clin Transplant 6:161-167

Ramos IM, Taylor KJM, Kier R, Burns PN, Snower DP & Carter D. (1988). Tumor vascular Signals in Renal Masses: Detection with Doppler US. Radiology. 168:633-637.

Rawashdeh YF, Mortensen J, Horlyck A, Olsen KO, Fisker RV, Schroll L & Frokiaer J. (2000). Resistive Index: an Experimental Study of Normal Range in the Pig. Scand J Urol Nephrol 34:10-14.

Rawashdeh YF, Djurhuus JC, Mortensen J, Horlyck A & Frokiaer J. (2001). The Intrarenal Resistive Index as Pathophysiologycal Marker of Obstructive Uropaty. J Urol 165: 1397-1404.

Riehl J, Schmitt H, Bongartz D, Bergmann D & Sieberth HG. (1997). Renal Artery Stenosis: Evaluation with Colour Duplex US. Nephrol Dial Transplant 12:1608-1614.

Rifkin MD, Needleman L & Pasto E. (1987). Evaluation of Renal Transplant Rejection by Duplex Doppler Examination: Value of the Resistive Index. Am J Roentgen 148:759-762.

Rigsby CM, Burns PN, Weltin GG, Chen B, Bia M & Taylor KJ. (1987). Doppler Signal Quantitation in Renal Allografts: Comparison in Normal and Rejecting Transplants with Pathologic Correlation. Radiology 162:239-242.

Rivers BJ, Walter PA & O'Brien TD. (1996). Duplex Doppler Estimation of Pourcelot Resistive Index in Arcuate Arteries of Sedated Normal Cats. J Vet Intern Med 10:28-33.

Rivers BJ, Walter PA, Polzin DJ & King VL. (1997a). Duplex Doppler Estimation of Intrarenal Pourcelot Resistive Index in Dogs And Cats with Renal Disease. J Vet Intern Med 11:250-260.

Rivers BJ, Walter PA, Letourneau JG, Finlay DE, Ritenour ER, King VL, O'Brien TD & Polzin DJ. (1997b). Duplex Doppler Estimation of Resistive Index in Arcuate Arteries of Sedated, Normal Female Dogs: Implications for Use in the Diagnosis of Renal Failure. J Am Anim Hosp Assoc. 33: 69-76.

Rodgers P, Bates J & Irving H. (1993). Intrarenal Doppler Ultrasound Studies in Normal and Acutely Obstructed Kidneys. Br J Radiol 65:207-212

Ruggenenti P, Mosconi L, Bruno S, Remuzzi A, Sangalli F, Lepre MS, Agazzi R, Nani R, Fasolini G & Remuzzi G. (2001). Post-transplant Renal Artery Stenosis: The Hemodynamic Response to Revascularization. Kidney Int 60:309-318.

Sari A, Dinc H, Zibandeh A, Telatar M & Gumele HR. (1999). Value of Resistive Index in Patients with Clinical Diabetic Nephropathy. Invest Radiol 34:718-721.

Scoble JE. (1999). Atherosclerotic Nephropathy. Kidney Int 56:106-109.

Schwerk WB, Restrepo IK, Stellwaag M, Klose KJ & Brittinger SC. (1994). Renal Artery Stenosis: Grading with Image-directed Doppler US Evaluation of Resistive Index. Radiology 190: 785-790.

Shimizu Y, Itoh T & Hougaku H. (2001). Clinical Usefulness of Duplex US for the Assessment of Renal Arteriosclerosis in Essential Hypertensive Patients. Hypertens Res 24:13-17.

Shokeir AA, Provoost AP, el-Azab M, Dawaba M & Nijman RJ. (1996). Renal Doppler Ultrasound in Children with Obstructive Uropathy: Effect of intravenous Normal Saline Fluid Load and Furosemide. J Urol 156:1455-1458.

Shokeir AA, Provoost AP & Nijman RJM. (1997a). Resistive Index in Obstructive Uropathy. Br J Urol 80;195-200.

Shokeir AA, Nijman RJM, El-Azab M & Provoost AP. (1997b). Partial Ureteral Obstruction: Role of Resistive Index in Stages of Obstruction and Release. Urology 49:528-535.

Shokeir AA, Abdulmaaboud M, Farage Y & Mutabagani H. (1999). Resistive Index in Renal Colic. The Effect of Nonsteroidal Anti-inflammatory Drugs. Br J Urol 84:249-51.

Shokeir AA & Abdulmaaboud M. (2001). Prospective Comparison of Nonenhanced Helical Computerized Tomography and Doppler US for the Diagnosis of Renal Colic. J Urol 165:1082-1084.

Sigirci A, Hallaç T, Akinci A, Temel I, Gülcan H, Aslan M, Koçer M, Kahraman B, Alkan A & Kutlu R. (2006). Renal Interlobar Artery Parameters with Duplex Doppler Sonography and Correlaions with Age, Plasma Renin, And Aldesterone Levels in Healthy Children. AJR 186:828-832.

Soldo D, Brkljacic B, Bozikov V, Drinkovic I & Hauser M. (1997). Diabetic Nephropathy: Comparison of Conventional and Duplex Doppler Ultrasonographic Findings. Acta Radiol 38:296-302.

Stavros AT, Parker SH, Yakes WF, Chantelois AE, Burke BJ, Meyers PR & Schenck JJ. (1992). Segmental Stenosis of the Renal Artery: Pattern Recognition of Tardus and Parvus Abnormalities with Duplex Sonography. Radiology 184:487-492.

Stavros AT & Harshfield D. (1994). Renal Doppler, Renal Artery Stenosis, and Renovascular Hypertension: Direct and Indirect Duplex Doppler Sonographic Abnormalities in Patients with Renal Artery Stenosis. Ultrasound Quarterly 12: 217-263.

Szatmari V, Sotonyi P & Vörös K. (2001). Normal Duplex Doppler Waveforms of the Major Abdominal Blood Vessels in Dogs. A Review. Vet Radiol Ultrasound 42:93-107.

Taylor KJW & Marks WH. (1990). Used Doppler Imaging for Evaluation of Dysfonction in Renal Allografts. AJR 155: 536-537.

Terry JD, Rysavy JA & Frick MP. (1992). Intrarenal Doppler: Characteristics of Aging Kidneys. J Ultrasound Med 11:647-651.

Tublin M, Dodd G & Verdile V. (1994). Acute Renal Colic: Diagnosis with Duplex Doppler US. Radiology 193:697-701.

Tublin ME, Tessler FN & Murphy ME. (1999). Correlation between Renal Vascular Resistance, Pulse Pressure, and the Resistive Index in Isolated Perfused Rabbit Kidneys. Radiology 213:258-264.

Tublin ME, Bude RO & Platt JF. (2003). Resistive Index in Renal Doppler Sonography: Where Do We Stand? AJR 180:885-892.

Trillaud H, Merville P, Linh PTL, Palussière J, Potaux L & Grenier N. (1998). Color Doppler Sonography in Early Renal Transplantation Follow-up: Resistive Index Measurements versus Power Doppler Sonography. AJR 171:1611-1615.

Ulrich JC, York JP & Koff SA. (1995). The Renal Vascular Response to Acutely Elevated Intrapelvic Pressure: Resistive Index Measurements in Experimental Urinary Obstruction. J Urol 154:1202-1204.

Vade A, Subbaiah P, Kalbhen CL & Ryva JC. (1993). Renal Resistive Indices in Children. J Ultrasound Med 12:655-658.

Wong SN, Lo RN & Yu EC. (1989). Renal Blood Flow Pattern by Noninvasive Doppler Ultrasound in Normal Children and Acute Renal Failure Patients. J Ultrasound Med 8:135-141.

Zubarev AV. (2001). Ultrasound of Renal Vessels. Eur Radiol 11:1902-1905.

2

Integrated Physiological Interaction Modeling and Simulation for Aerobic Circulation with Beat-by-Beat Hemodynamics

Kenichi Asami and Mochimitsu Komori
Kyushu Institute of Technology
Japan

1. Introduction

This chapter describes a simulation system for modeling and testing aerobic circulatory physiology on the virtual environment. There have been many models of the biological system at various scales and from various viewpoints, intended to simulate physiological changes and pathological conditions (McLeod, 1966). However, these models are designed primarily for medical education, and are unsuitable as practical tools for clinical diagnosis. The reason for this unsuitability is their insufficiently accurate quantitative representation of the physiological system compared to clinical data or the results of animal experiments (Ackerman, 1991). A further problem in developing practically useful models of biological systems is the need for expert physiologists to engage in computer programming in order to create the mathematical models. The useful modeling and simulation tool for an integrated circulatory system is important for physiological diagnosis and evaluation.

The development of a simulation tool that uses a basic exercise model of circulatory system enables to facilitate model testing, formulation, and refinement for solving the above problems. Another purpose is to provide a basic model that combines macro and micro models for the aerobic circulation with the heart function. The macro model includes the comprehensive physiological functions, and the micro model analyzes the pulsatile behavior of the hemodynamics in adaptive fitness support. By combining the macro and micro models of the circulatory system, it becomes possible to simulate subtle changes of the blood flow in response to various factors, such as body temperature, body weight, and basic metabolism, which is impossible using a single-purpose model.

In this simulation system, the macro model includes multiple organs and physiological functions, and calculates the physiological variables with time steps of a second or longer. The macro model is designed to allow the calculation of long-term biological phenomena over periods ranging from several hours to several months. In the heart activity, on the other hand, time steps of the order of milliseconds or microseconds are required in order to analyze the contraction and expansion cycle of the heart, which takes place in a cardiac period of less than a second. Consequently, the micro model is designed to calculate variables with a time step of less than a second, focusing on a single physiological function.

The integrated physiological simulation would be proposed, here a basic model that combines the macro and micro models of the aerobic circulatory system is provided. In addition, a modeling support function is proposed in which sensitivity analysis is used to assist the user in modifying the basic model. In an experiment using the combined macro and micro model, realistic simulation results were obtained for the blood flow, lactic mass, and O_2 consumption when the parameters representing the exercise intensity was varied.

2. Circulatory system model

The macro model of the circulatory system comprehensively describes multiple organs and physiological functions. The circulatory system model (Coleman, 1979; Randall, 1987) includes 25 physiological modules, including 321 variables and 70 parameters. The 25 modules are as follows: *HEART* (cardiac output and blood flow to major organs), *CARDFUNC* (strength levels of left and right heart), *CIRC* (pulmonary circulation), *REFLEX-1* and *REFLEX-2* (the activities of sympathetic nerve and vagus nerve, and heart rate), *TEMP* (heat generation and consumption in body temperature), *EXER* (control of exercise), *DRUGS* (prescription of drugs), O_2 (oxygen balance), CO_2 (carbon dioxide balance), *VENT* (control of ventilation), *GAS* (gas exchange), *HORMONES* (hormone adjustment), *KIDNEY* (kidney function and status), *RENEX* (excretion from kidneys), *HEMOD* (hemodialysis), *FLUIDS* (injection and loss of systemic fluids), *WATER* (water balance), *NA* (sodium balance), *ACID/BASE* (acid-base balance), *UREA* (urine balance), *K* (potassium balance), *PROTEIN* (protein balance), *VOLUMES* (blood distribution), and *BLOOD* (hematocrit control), which are connected with input and output variables shown in Fig. 1.

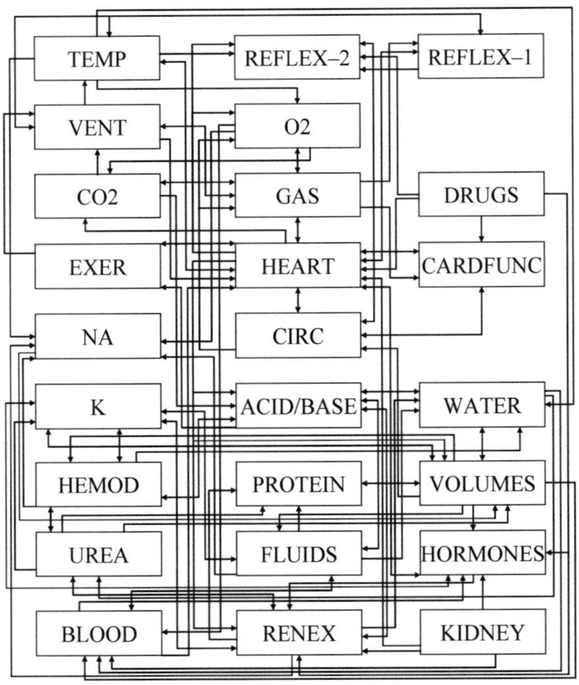

Fig. 1. Modules connected with input and output variables

2.1 Sensitivity analysis

The proposed simulation system provides the user with the ability to modify the basic macro model. The user could wish to examine the quantitative behavior of the output variables by simulation, and to correct the time course of the output variables. It is necessary in such cases to trace the input variable and the parameters that strongly affect the output variables under consideration. The modeling support is a function that helps such tracing of variables. It can be utilized effectively to view the structure of the mathematical expressions in the module. The modeling support function applies sensitivity analysis to the module. The sensitivities among the variables are represented by a directed graph that visualizes the causal relations among variables. The directed graph has a hierarchical structure, indicating the extent to which output variables are affected by individual input variables or parameters. By using this function, the user can determine which parameters should be adjusted and by how much in order to move the output variable toward the target value.

Fig. 2 outlines the sensitivity analysis of a simple module. *I* denotes an input variable, *O* an output variable, *M* an intermediate variable used for convenience in computation, and *P* a parameter. In this study, sensitivity is defined as the ratio of the rate of change of the output variable to the rate of change of the input variable in the module. In sensitivity analysis, the value of the input variable is temporarily increased by 10%, and the percentage in output variable changes is determined. A simple example is presented below. Consider the computation formula $A = B + 2*C$. From this formula, the two causal relations $B \rightarrow A$ (sensitivity 0.333) and $C \rightarrow A$ (sensitivity 0.666) are derived as paths in the directed graph. The sensitivities are calculated by setting the initial values of both *B* and *C* to 100. The sensitivity to parameters is similarly determined. When the directed graph contains an intermediate variable, the sensitivities are calculated for the two paths passing through the intermediate variable. Then the paths are replaced by a path corresponding to the product, and the intermediate variable is eliminated. However, it may happen that an output variable is also used as an intermediate variable. The output variable has the role of describing the

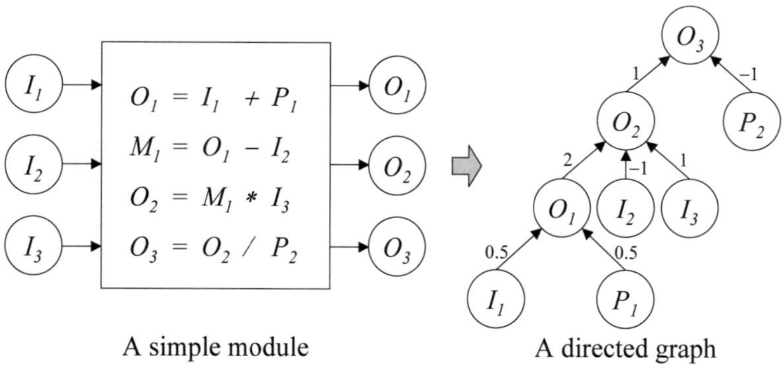

I: input *O*: output *P*: parameter *M*: medium variable

Definition:

$$Sensitivity = \frac{\Delta Rate\ of\ Output}{\Delta Rate\ of\ Input}$$

Calculation:

$$Sensitivity = \frac{O'-O}{O} \Big/ \frac{I'-I}{I}$$

Fig. 2. Outline of sensitivity analysis

behavior of the module and is not eliminated, since it must be referred to by other modules. In the directed graph shown in Fig. 2, there are seven causal relations ($I_1 \rightarrow O_1$, $P_1 \rightarrow O_1$, $I_2 \rightarrow O_2$, $O_1 \rightarrow O_2$, $I_3 \rightarrow O_2$, $O_2 \rightarrow O_3$, $P_2 \rightarrow O_3$) among the variables. In this case, the sensitivity is calculated by setting the initial values of all the input variables and parameter values to 100. The modeling support is a function that helps the user to understand the causal relations among the variables. It traces the parameters, starting from the output variable, and finally identifies the parameter that most strongly affects the output variable of accompanying with the sensitivity. Suppose that the user wishes to modify the value of output variable O_3. The user then traces the path among the variables, $P_1 \rightarrow O_1 \rightarrow O_2 \rightarrow O_3$, in the editorial interface and ascertains the sensitivity of parameter P_1 for the output variable O_3. The user can then correct the behavior of the output variable by adjusting the parameter value.

2.2 Structural analysis

The structure of equations, variables, and parameters of module is visualized to the hierarchy by the ISM (Interpretive Structural Modeling). Because the directed graph consisting of extracted linkages does not explain the whole systematic order of cause-effect relationships, a user would not be able to grasp how to calculate an output variable from other input variables and parameters. The structural analysis by ISM classifies variables and parameters in accordance with the hierarchical levels, which are obtained by finding a set of nodes that cannot reach any other nodes except the set itself. The hierarchized directed graph guarantees that only the linkages from the lower level to the upper level are included in the whole graph, but there is no reverse directional one. Nodes in the same level means to be either irrelevant to each other or related mutually. The structure of causal relationships among variables and parameters enables the simulation system to solve effectively a diagnostic problem, which is defined as follows: An output variable whose value is out of its normal range is given, all input variables which can reach to the output are found into the hierarchical graph, and an input variable whose path to the output has the maximum total gain is proposed as a causative one for adjusting the unusual output's value. Otherwise parameter is considered as causative factor in the abnormal variation of the output. The total gain helps to decide major causative inputs and parameters because the maximum gain says that they can be the most noteworthy factors about the change of the output.

Fig.3 shows the hierarchy of the module *ACID/BASE*, where acidity in blood is determined. Here variables figured by square and parameters by ellipse are classified to 6 levels. There are two final output variables *PH* (blood pH) in the top level and *BICARB* (plasma bicarbonate) in the 3rd level. They clearly depend on other variables and parameters in the lower levels. The module *ACID/BASE* contains input variables PCO_2 (venous CO_2 tension) from module CO_2, *BICRT* (added bicarbonate) from module *FLUIDS*, *EXBIC* (excretion of bicarbonate) from module *RENEX*, *DYBIC* (dialyzed bicarbonate), BH_2OL (body water in litters) from module *WATER*, and DMO_2C (delta muscle O_2) from module *HEART*, and has one parameter *BACID* (basic acid production), which are terminal nodes of this module. It is visualized that there are well-ordered connections of variables, such as *BICRT* → *DBIM* → *BIMASS* → *BICARB*, from input to output in the module. Fig.4 describes the hierarchy classified in 6 levels of module *BLOOD*, where blood volume and red cell mass are calculated. The outputs are *HCT* (hematocrit), *BV* (blood volume), and *WGHT* (body weight). *WGHT* is calculated from parameter *OBM* (other body mass), input BH_2OL (body water in litters) from module *WATER*, and variable *RCM* (red cell mass). The hierarchical directed graphs not only help to understand the calculation structure of the module, but also enable to track paths between input and output variables that are connected with recursive links in the large circulatory system model. Exploring large structure of cause and effect relationships becomes effective with respect to diagnosis time by ignoring irrelevant paths among input and output variables.

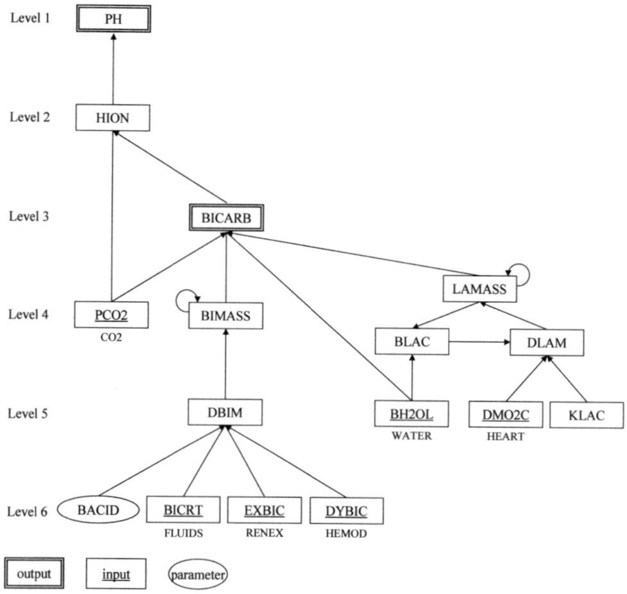

Fig. 3. Hierarchical directed graph of module *ACID/BASE*

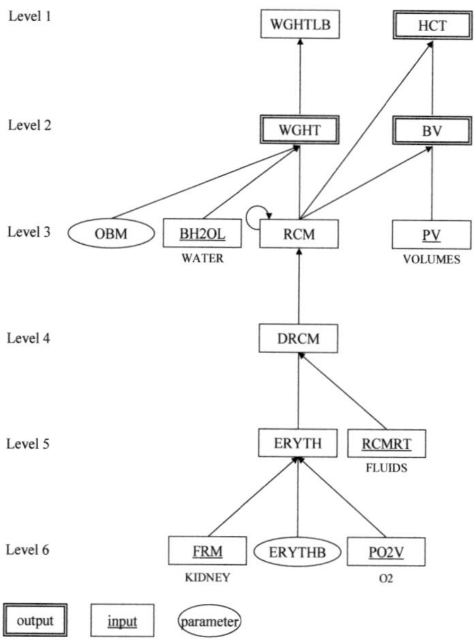

Fig. 4. Hierarchical directed graph of module *BLOOD*

3. Beat-by-beat model

The hemodynamics of the heart as a pump could be described as a micro model based on time-varying elasticity from the Frank-Starling law, which defines the ventricular mechanical properties in a cardiac cycle. The *HEART* module simulates hemodynamics in the macro model with the aortic pressure, the cardiac output, and the blood flow to the major organs. However, it is a macroscopic model, and the pulsations cannot be represented even if the time step of temporal changes is shortened to millisecond order. Therefore, a micro model of the circulatory system is constructed so that hemodynamics with periodic pulsations due to heart activity can be simulated. The definition of ventricular elastance as the ratio of ventricular pressure to volume indicates, $E_v(t) = P_v(t)/(V_v(t)-V_0)$ where the inferior v refers to the ventricle and V_0 represents the unstressed volume of ventricles. Fig. 5 shows the function of the time-varying elastance, which repeats systole and diastole for ejecting blood from the chamber. During the systolic phase of the ventricle, elastance rises rapidly, and the rise ceases at ejection. During the diastolic phase of the ventricle, elastance falls rapidly in isovolumetric relaxation, and is almost constant in passive filling.

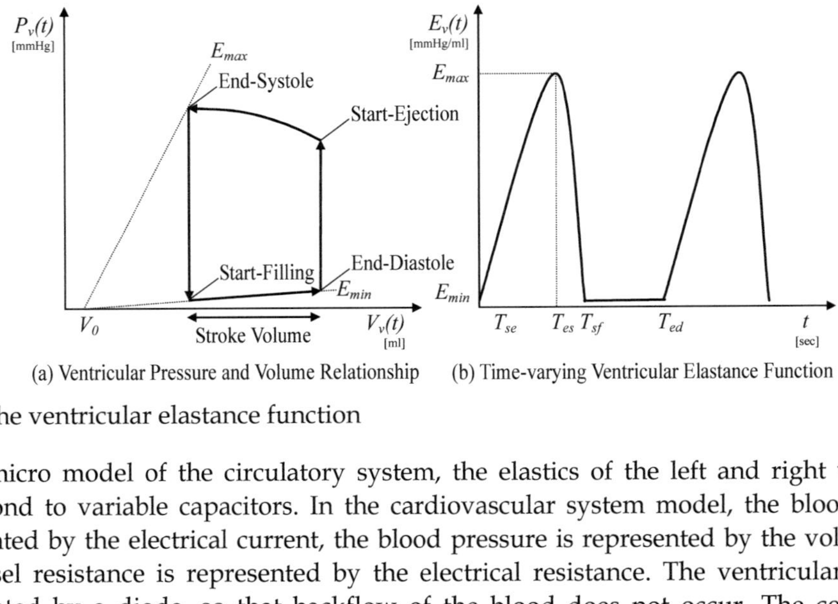

(a) Ventricular Pressure and Volume Relationship (b) Time-varying Ventricular Elastance Function

Fig. 5. The ventricular elastance function

In the micro model of the circulatory system, the elastics of the left and right ventricles correspond to variable capacitors. In the cardiovascular system model, the blood flow is represented by the electrical current, the blood pressure is represented by the voltage, and the vessel resistance is represented by the electrical resistance. The ventricular valve is represented by a diode, so that backflow of the blood does not occur. The compliance simulates the softness of the vessels and the blood pool in the vessels, and corresponds to the capacitor in the electrical circuit. Fig. 6 shows the electrical circuit model of systemic circulation, and Fig. 7 pulmonary circulation. The systemic and pulmonary circulation is closed in series by connecting points A and B. The aortic flow output from the left ventricle (Q_{ao}) branches into the brain vessel blood flow (Q_{br}), the coronary vessel blood flow (Q_{co}), the renal vessel blood flow (Q_{re}), the skin vessel blood flow (Q_{sk}), the muscle vessel blood flow (Q_{mu}), the bronchial vessel flow (Q_{bc}), and the other vessel blood flow (Q_{ot}). On their return, the blood flows are combined in the vena cava and the right atrium to form the right ventricular blood flow (Q_{rv}). The outlet valve is the aortic valve and the inlet valve is the mitral valve. Compliances are provided with the systemic artery compliance C_{sa} and the systemic vein and right atrium compliance C_{sv}. Three differential equations are derived from

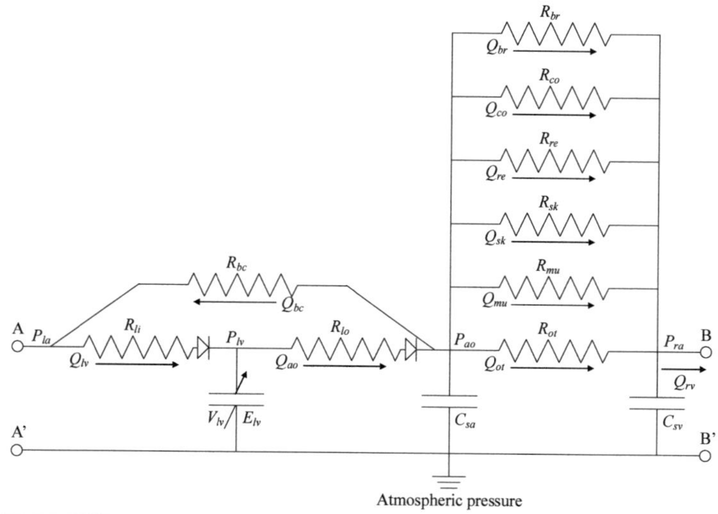

P_{lv} : Pressure in left ventricle [mmHg]	E_{lv} : Elastance of left ventricle [mmHg/ml]
P_{la} : Pressure in left atrium [mmHg]	V_{lv} : Volume of left ventricle [ml]
P_{ao} : Pressure in aorta [mmHg]	C_{sa} : Compliance of systemic artery [ml/mmHg]
	C_{sv} : Compliance of systemic vein and right atrium [ml/mmHg]
Q_{lv} : Quantity to left ventricle [ml/sec]	R_{li} : Resistance of left ventricular inflow valve [mmHg/ml/sec]
Q_{ao}: Quantity to aorta [ml/sec]	R_{lo} : Resistance of left ventricular outflow valve [mmHg/ml/sec]
Q_{br} : Quantity to brain blood vessel [ml/sec]	R_{br} : Resistance of brain blood vessel [mmHg/ml/sec]
Q_{bc} : Quantity to bronchial blood vessel [ml/sec]	R_{bc} : Resistance of bronchial blood vessel [mmHg/ml/sec]
Q_{co} : Quantity to coronary blood vessel [ml/sec]	R_{co} : Resistance of coronary blood vessel [mmHg/ml/sec]
Q_{re} : Quantity to renal blood vessel [ml/sec]	R_{re} : Resistance of renal blood vessel [mmHg/ml/sec]
Q_{sk} : Quantity to skin blood vessel [ml/sec]	R_{sk} : Resistance of skin blood vessel [mmHg/ml/sec]
Q_{mu}: Quantity to muscle blood vessel [ml/sec]	R_{mu}: Resistance of muscle blood vessel [mmHg/ml/sec]
Q_{ot} : Quantity to other blood vessel [ml/sec]	R_{ot} : Resistance of other blood vessel [mmHg/ml/sec]

Fig. 6. The systemic circulation model

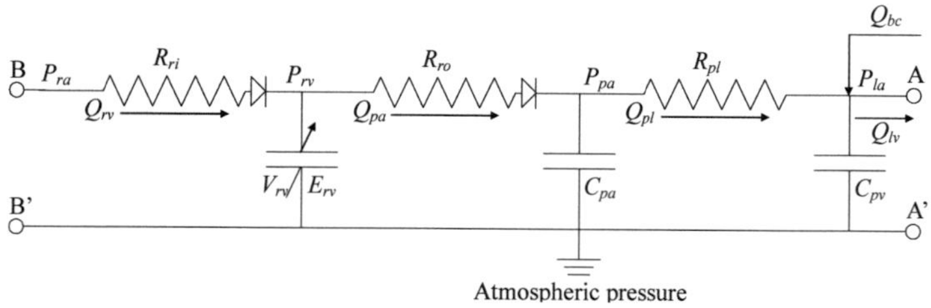

P_{rv} : Pressure in right ventricle [mmHg]	E_{rv} : Elastance of right ventricle [mmHg/ml]
P_{ra} : Pressure in right atrium [mmHg]	V_{rv} : Volume of right ventricle [ml]
P_{pa} : Pressure in pulmonary artery [mmHg]	C_{pa} : Compliance of pulmonary artery [ml/mmHg]
	C_{pv} : Compliance of pulmonary vein and left atrium [ml/mmHg]
Q_{rv} : Quantity to right ventricle [ml/sec]	R_{ri} : Resistance of right ventricular inflow valve [mmHg/ml/sec]
Q_{pa} : Quantity to pulmonary artery [ml/sec]	R_{ro} : Resistance of right ventricular outflow valve [mmHg/ml/sec]
Q_{pl} : Quantity to pulmonary blood vessel[ml/sec]	R_{pl} : Resistance of pulmonary blood vessel [mmHg/ml/sec]

Fig. 7. The pulmonary circulation model

the electrical circuit model of the systemic circulation, based on the relations among the changes in blood flows. Equations (1), (2), and (3) are concerned with the changes of the blood flow in the left ventricle, the aorta, and the vena cava, respectively. Three variables, namely, the left ventricular volume V_{lv}, the aortic pressure P_{ao}, and the right atrium pressure P_{ra}, are described by the differential equations:

$$\frac{dV_{lv}}{dt} = Q_{lv} - Q_{ao} \tag{1}$$

$$\frac{dP_{ao}}{dt} = \frac{Q_{ao} - Q_{br} - Q_{co} - Q_{re} - Q_{sk} - Q_{mu} - Q_{ot} - Q_{bc}}{C_{sa}} \tag{2}$$

$$\frac{dP_{ra}}{dt} = \frac{Q_{br} + Q_{co} + Q_{re} + Q_{sk} + Q_{mu} + Q_{ot} - Q_{rv}}{C_{sv}} \tag{3}$$

The left ventricular pressure P_{lv} can be determined based on the relation among the pressure, the volume, and the elastance of the left ventricle. Here E_{lv} is the elastance, V_{lv} is the volume, and V_{lv0} is the unloaded volume, respectively, of the left ventricle:

$$P_{lv} = E_{lv} \times (V_{lv} - V_{lv0}) \tag{4}$$

The blood flow into the left ventricle (Q_{lv}) and the blood flow from the left ventricle (Q_{ao}) can be determined by Ohm's law from the change in the blood pressure and the vessel resistance. Since a valve is present, no backflow occurs in the inlet and outlet blood flows of the left ventricle:

$$Q_{lv} = \begin{cases} \dfrac{P_{la} - P_{lv}}{R_{li}} & if \quad P_{la} > P_{lv} \\ 0 & if \quad P_{la} \le P_{lv} \end{cases} \tag{5}$$

$$Q_{ao} = \begin{cases} \dfrac{P_{lv} - P_{ao}}{R_{lo}} & if \quad P_{lv} > P_{ao} \\ 0 & if \quad P_{lv} \le P_{ao} \end{cases} \tag{6}$$

The blood flow to each vessel in the systemic circulation system can be similarly determined from the change in the blood pressure and the vessel resistance. For example, the blood flow in the brain vessel is calculated as follows:

$$Q_{br} = \frac{P_{ao} - P_{ra}}{R_{br}} \tag{7}$$

The pulmonary arterial flow (Q_{pa}) output from the right ventricle flows in the pulmonary vessel (Q_{pl}) to the pulmonary vein and left atrium, and then into the left ventricle (Q_{lv}). The outlet valve is the pulmonary valve, and the inlet valve is the tricuspid valve. Compliances are provided with the pulmonary artery compliance C_{pa} and the pulmonary vein and left atrium compliance C_{pv}. The following three differential equations are derived from the change in blood flow in the electrical circuit model of the pulmonary circulation. Equations (8), (9), and (10) are concerned with the blood flows in the right ventricle, the pulmonary artery, and the pulmonary vein, respectively. Three variables, the right ventricular volume V_{rv}, the pulmonary artery pressure P_{pa}, and the left atrium pressure P_{la}, are described by the differential equations:

$$\frac{dV_{rv}}{dt} = Q_{rv} - Q_{pa} \tag{8}$$

$$\frac{dP_{pa}}{dt} = \frac{Q_{pa} - Q_{pl}}{C_{pa}} \tag{9}$$

$$\frac{dP_{la}}{dt} = \frac{Q_{pl} + Q_{bc} - Q_{lv}}{C_{pv}} \tag{10}$$

The right ventricular pressure P_{rv} can be determined similarly. Here E_{rv} is the elastance, V_{rv} is the volume, and V_{rv0} is the unloaded volume, respectively, of the right ventricle:

$$P_{rv} = E_{rv} \times (V_{rv} - V_{rv0}) \tag{11}$$

The blood flow into the right ventricle (Q_{rv}) and the blood flow from the right ventricle (Q_{pa}) can be determined from the change in the blood pressure and the vessel resistance:

$$Q_{rv} = \begin{cases} \dfrac{P_{ra} - P_{rv}}{R_{ri}} & if \quad P_{ra} > P_{rv} \\ 0 & if \quad P_{ra} \le P_{rv} \end{cases} \tag{12}$$

$$Q_{pa} = \begin{cases} \dfrac{P_{rv} - P_{pa}}{R_{ro}} & if \quad P_{rv} > P_{pa} \\ 0 & if \quad P_{rv} \le P_{pa} \end{cases} \tag{13}$$

The blood flow in the pulmonary vessel (Q_{pl}) is calculated similarly:

$$Q_{pl} = \frac{P_{pa} - P_{la}}{R_{pl}} \tag{14}$$

The cardiovascular system model consisting of systemic and pulmonary circulations is connected to the basic macro model with common variables of vascular resistance, heart rate, and body weight. Moreover, the cardiovascular system model products beat-by-beat blood flow and pressure as output. Numerical analysis using the Runge-Kutta-Gill method aiming at high speed calculation is applied to the differential equations (1) to (14). The micro model of the circulatory system is written in C programming language to take priority on the computation speed in the simulation.

4. Exercise control model

A suitable exercise level is presented and controlled according to the individual hemodynamic conditions. The responses of respiration, venous contraction, and muscle metabolism for exercise are presented in the circulatory system model. The exercise is defined as the addition of oxygen in blood from 0 to 10,000 ml/min for normal oxygen use 250 ml/min. Fig. 8 shows basic relationships between physiological variables in the exercise control model. If the exercise is given, respiration rate, sympathetic activity, venous pressure, and muscular metabolism increase according to the exercise levels. Consequently, cardiac output and venous return rise in the circulatory system. In addition to the above functions, the exercise control model is constructed by introducing personal parameters of body weight, height, age, and sex and evaluation variables of maximum oxygen uptake, basal metabolic rate, and body fat percentage, related to fitness training. By giving personal parameters, the simulation system could calculate adequate exercise levels. In the exercise control model, actual exercise intensity, ventilation in exercise, and venous multiplier in exercise are calculated. Here, the exercise is terminated if blood pH becomes 7 or less acidity, consciousness is lost, oxygen debt exceeds 10 l/min, or coronary ischemia happens.

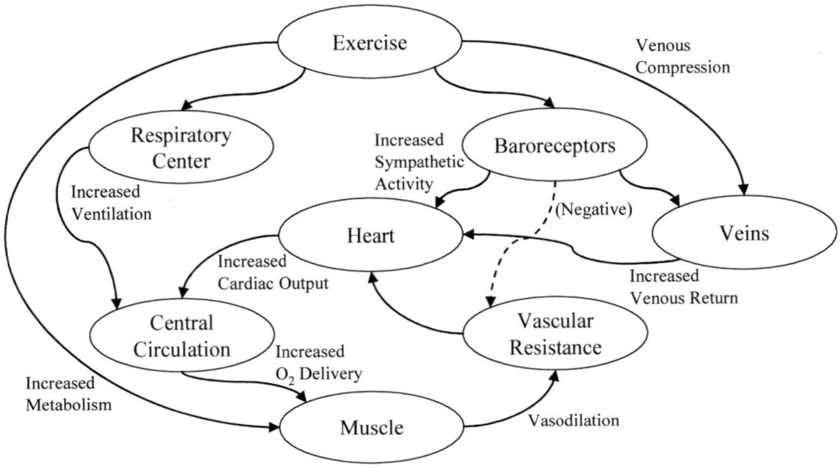

Fig. 8. The relationship among variables in exercise control model

VO_2max as exercise intensity promotes individual endurance and performance. Understanding personal *VO_2max* in ml/kg/min or aerobic power is the key for enhancing personal maximum uptake of oxygen, because it indicates the maximum amount of oxygen the person can take in and utilize. The exercise control model uses *VO_2max* for deciding when the fitness training should be terminated, although the amount of oxygen debt does not reach to 10,000 ml/min. *VO_2max* is described as the following equation by Wolthuis depending on the age, gender, and fitness habits, where the first coefficient is set to 50.6 for the active level, 45.8 for the moderate level and 43.2 for the sedentary level. For women, the value becomes 75% regardless of age. Thus the maximum oxygen uptake is determined by multiplying *VO_2max* by body weight.

$$VO_2max = 50.6 - 0.17 \times AGE \tag{15}$$

Basal metabolic rate (*BMR*) is an estimate of how many calories the body would burn if the person was to do nothing but rest for 24 hours. It represents the minimal amount of caloric requirement needed to sustain life including heart beating, lungs breathing, and body temperature normal in a resting individual. The purposes of the fitness training would be health and weight management in many cases. Therefore, *BMR* is an essential index in the exercise control model, and influences to calorie production presented to the user. *BMR* is calculated by the Harris-Benedict equation from weight in kilograms, height in centimeters, and age in years, where the upper one is used for men and the lower for women.

$$\begin{cases} BMR = 66 + (13.75 \times WEIGHT) + (5.0 \times HEIGHT) - (6.76 \times AGE) \\ BMR = 655 + (9.56 \times WEIGHT) + (1.85 \times HEIGHT) - (4.68 \times AGE) \end{cases} \quad (16)$$

Body composition and health are affected by the amount of body fat because muscle tissue is more compact than fat. Measuring changes in body fat percentage, rather than just measuring changes in weight, can be very motivational for dieting. Body fat percentage is measured by several methods, such as bioelectrical impedance, skin fold measurement, hydrostatic weighing, and infrared interactance. In the exercise control model, body fat percentage as input influences to muscle mobilizing rate in the fitness training.

5. Simulation results

The macro and micro models of the circulatory system are combined through the common variables. It is important to synthesize the macro model with comprehensive parameters and the micro model with beat-by-beat hemodynamics for evaluating fitness support. The inputs from the macro model to the micro model are the vessel resistance, the heart rate, and the body weight. The outputs from the micro model are the blood pressure and the blood flow for the major vascular parts. By combining the macro and micro models, it becomes possible to simulate microscopics in hemodynamics that are affected by the parameters of the whole body. After a step (default 15 seconds) is performed in the macro model, the values of the vessel resistance in each subsystem are passed to the micro model. Then, the micro model runs for 15 seconds (with a default step of 0.01 second), and the 15-second average values of the blood flow in each component and of the aortic flow (Q_{ao}) and aortic pressure (P_{ao}) are passed to the macro model.

5.1 Simulation for body weight

Using the integrated macro and micro models, we confirmed whether a quantitatively adequate result could be obtained by the simulation when the body weight parameter was varied. Three values of the body weight parameter were input, namely, 50, 65, and 80 kg. Fig. 9 shows the simulation results of the aortic flow for various body weight parameters. The waveform is shown for 5 seconds after the steady state is reached. The micro mode required approximately 10 seconds until steady state for the blood flow was reached. The average aortic flow for a pulsation cycle is 4997 ml/min for a body weight of 50 kg, 6384 ml/min for 65 kg, and 7719 ml/min for 80 kg. We see that the aortic flow increases roughly in proportion to the body weight and that the average as a function of the body weight changes as approximately 100 ml/kg/min. The average aortic pressure is 99 mmHg for a body weight of 50 kg, 97 mmHg for 65 kg, and 96 mmHg for 80 kg. Thus, the aortic pressure is approximately 100 mmHg and remains almost constant independently of the body weight. The result for the blood flow is similar for vessels other than the aorta. Thus, the adequate pulsatile hemodynamics can be observed, which is impossible if only the macro model is used. The hemodynamic results obtained by the micro model are quantitatively reasonable as the body weight parameter is varied.

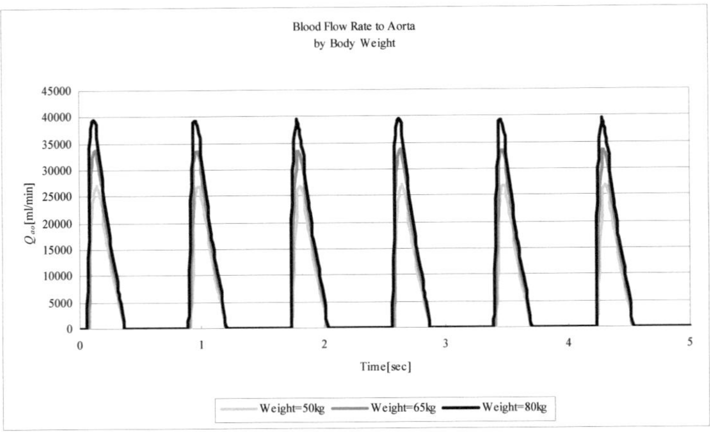

Fig. 9. Micro changes in aortic blood flow by body weight

5.2 Simulation for ambient temperature

We investigated whether a quantitatively adequate result could be obtained by the simulation when the ambient temperature parameter was varied. Because it is impossible to evaluate physical condition under considerable bad environment by subjects, the simulation system contributes to find the hemodynamic behavior for experimental approach in fitness support. The ambient temperature parameter (*TEMAB*) was raised by 10 °C and 20 °C from the initial value of 27 °C. In the macro model, the body temperature (*TEMP*) is described by an integral function of heat generation and loss. Heat generation depends on metabolism, exercise, and shivering. Heat loss depends on skin blood flow, perspiration, ambient temperature, and moisture. Fig. 10 shows the simulation result for microscopic changes of the skin blood flow for various ambient temperatures. The figure shows the time course of the change in the period from 5 seconds to 1 hour after the start of the simulation, when the skin blood flow reaches a steady state. The average skin blood flow for a pulsation is 377 ml/min for an ambient temperature of 27 °C, 640 ml/min for 37 °C, and 802 ml/min for 47 °C. The heart rate is 72 for an ambient temperature of 27 °C, 79 for 37 °C, and 83 for 47 °C.

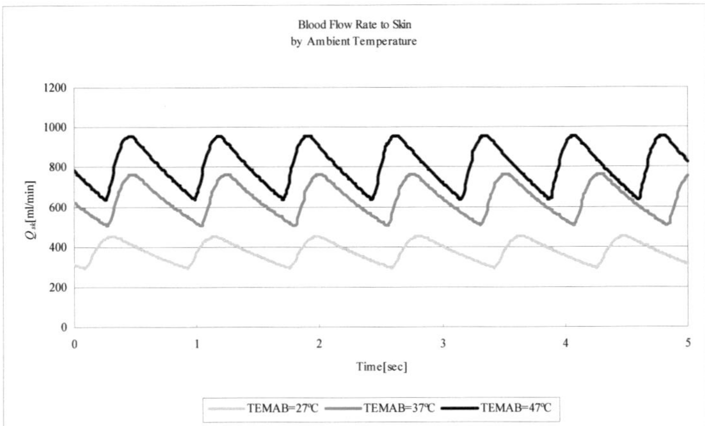

Fig. 10. Micro changes in skin blood flow by ambient temperature

Thus, the heart rate increases with the ambient temperature. By coupling the macro and micro models, it becomes possible to observe both the macro and micro aspects of changes. When the ambient temperature parameter is changed, the blood flow in the skin and in other vessels is obtained as a realistic value. Using this simulation system, the hemodynamics can be examined when the ambient temperature is raised to 47 °C, which is not easy to determine in real subjects.

5.3 Simulation for exercise load intensity

The parameter of gradual exercise load intensity of 100W, 200W, and 300W was introduced to the integrated circulatory system model. The parameter of exercise intensity was introduced to the macro model of the circulatory system, in which hemodynamic, respiratory, metabolismic, and sympathetic activities would increase. It was confirmed that evaluation of exercise for setting up an optimum load could be expressed by the model. Personal parameters with body weight of 60kg, height of 175cm, age of 40 years old, the male sex, body fat percentage of 20%, and fitness habit of the moderate level were set in this exercise evaluation. 2 hours of a continuous exercise and subsequent 1 hour of a steady state were given to the model.

Fig. 11 and 12 show the simulation results for physiological variables related to the exercise evaluation. Lactic acid is produced by anaerobic metabolism mainly from muscles, and it can be used as an index of the intensity of exercise training. Moreover, lactic acid production is proportional to oxygen debt. In Fig. 11, lactate mass rapidly went up to 250 mmol when the exercise intensity was set to 300W. Generally, produced lactic acid is used as energy to a certain amount of exercise intensity. In Fig. 12, Muscle O_2 use was almost proportional to the exercise intensity, where the marginal exercise intensity could be determined by being kept muscle O_2 use less than VO_2max.

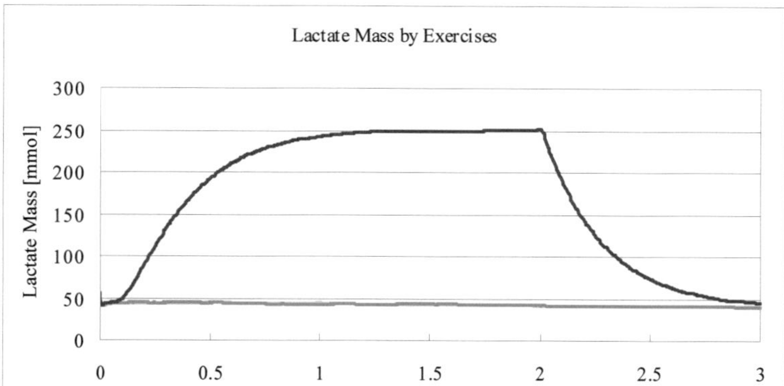

Fig. 11. Macro changes in lactate mass by exercise load intensity

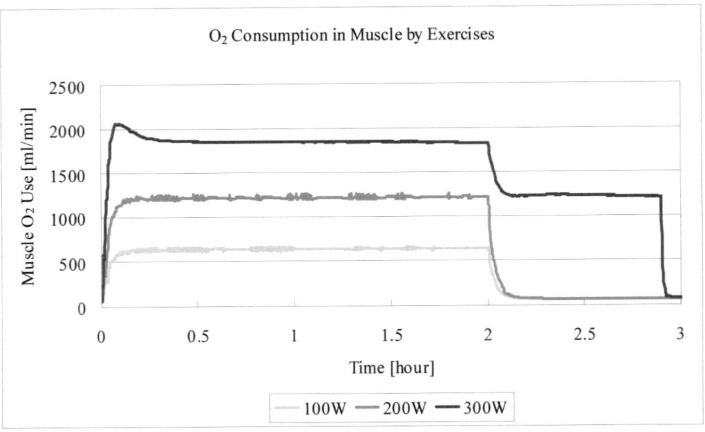

Fig. 12. Macro changes in O_2 consumption in muscle by exercise load intensity

Fig. 13 and 14 show the simulation results for blood flow to muscle and skin in an aerobic state of 5 seconds by the cardiovascular system model according to exercise intensities of 100W, 200W, and 300W. The muscle blood flow (Q_{mu}) was 5649 ml/min for 100W, 9648 ml/min for 200W, and 12520 ml/min for 300W. The skin blood flow (Q_{sk}) was 849 ml/min for 100W, 1063 ml/min for 200W, and 1509 ml/min for 300W. Moreover, the cardiac output (Q_{ao}) was 10435 ml/min for 100W, 14295 ml/min for 200W, and 17146 ml/min for 300W. The heart rate rose 87 for 100W, 102 for 200W, and 121 for 300W. In a resting condition, about 25% of cardiac output flows to muscle and skin. In an exercising condition, about 85% of cardiac output flows to muscle and skin. In Fig. 13 and 14, 62% of cardiac output for 100W, 74% of cardiac output for 200W, and 82% for cardiac output for 300W flowed to muscle and skin in the cardiovascular system model. By this exercise evaluation, the macro and micro behavior of blood flow control were adequate in the duration of 2 hours that the respective exercise load intensity was given and on the post exercise condition of 1 hour. Basically, the ratio of blood vessel resistances for muscle and skin decreased by the exercise control and the temperature regulation functions, and the heart rate increased by the sympathetic nerve activity and the cardiac output control functions. Consequently, the micro hemodynamics was quantitatively reasonable on the exercise conditions.

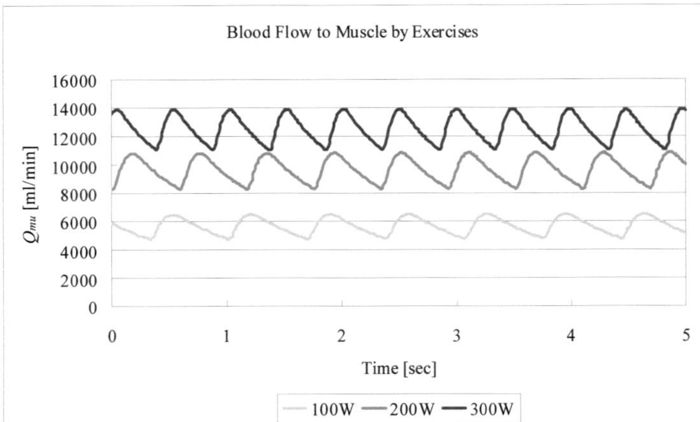

Fig. 13. Micro changes in muscle blood flow by exercise load intensity

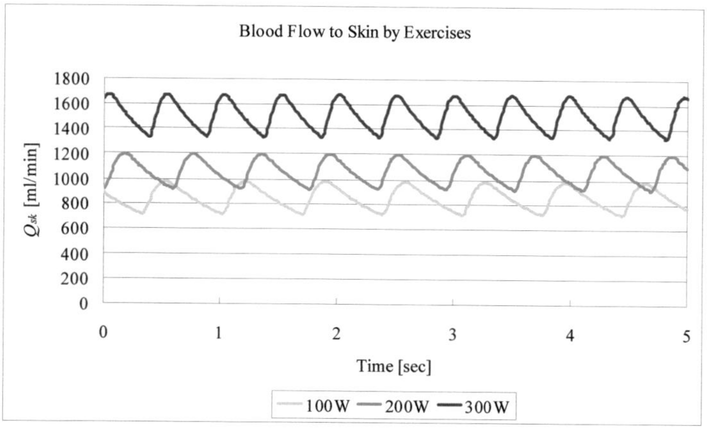

Fig. 14. Micro changes in skin blood flow by exercise load intensity

6. Conclusion

This chapter described a simulation system which combines macro and micro models of the circulatory system for exercise evaluation. In the simulation system, a macro model which includes multiple organs and functions and a micro model which describes a single physiological function are connected to provide the basic model. It is expected that the simulation system using integrated macro and micro models would be useful for comprehensive understanding of the physiological interactions for fitness support.

The proposed modeling support function can trace the sensitivities among the variables and parameters in the physiological modules. When part of a large-scale physiological model is modified, it may happen that the temporal behavior of the output variable changes greatly. In order to handle such situations, the user can examine the sensitivities of the output variables to each parameter, rather than performing many repeated simulations, and the adjustment of parameter values and the modification of the mathematical formulas can be systematically achieved.

Remaining problems include spatial refinement of the micro model in the cardiovascular system model. In the present micro model, only the blood flow branching into major vessels has been constructed. The compliance, which represents the elasticity of the vessels and the blood reservoir in the vessels, is taken into account at only four points. It is planned to refine the vessel system down to parts other than the capillaries by using anatomical data in order to allow simulations for the evaluation of detailed O_2 consumption in muscle. In order to apply the fitness support for practical use, the technological development to measure more precise physiological data would be need. Detailed dynamic data for O_2/CO_2 and lactic acid concentration in blood are essential to the extension of the exercise control model. The sensitivities and the hierarchized directed graph of the exercise control model need to be sophisticated so that the diagnosis and evaluation of aerobic hemodynamics could help efficiently fitness activity under various situations.

7. Acknowledgment

This study was supported in part by a Grant-in-Aid for Scientific Research (C) (KAKENHI 20560387) from the Ministry of Education, Culture, Sports, Science, and Technology of Japan.

8. References

Ackerman, M.J. (1991). The Visible Human Project, *Journal of Biocommunication*, vol.18, no.2, p.14

Coleman, T.G. (1979). A Mathematical Model for the Human Body in Health, Disease, and during Treatment, *ISA Transactions*, vol.18, no.3, pp.65-73

Hunter, P.J. (1999). Integrative Physiology of the Heart: The Development of Anatomically and Biophysically Based Mathematical Models of Myocardial Activation, Cardiac Mechanics and Coronary Flow, *Proceedings of the 47th Annual Scientific Meeting of the Cardiac Society of Australia and New Zealand*, Wellington, pp.7-11

Johnson, C.; Parker, S.; Hansen, C.; Kindlmann, G. & Livnat, Y. (1999). Interactive Simulation and Visualization, *IEEE Computer*, vol.32, no.12, pp.59-65

McLeod, J. (1966). PHYSBE: A Physiological Simulation Benchmark Experiment, *Simulation*, vol.7, no.6, pp.324-329

Noble, D. (2002). Modeling the Heart - from Genes to Cells to the Whole Organ, *Science*, vol.295, pp.1678-1682

Randall, J.E. (1987). *Microcomputers and Physiological Simulation*, Raven, New York

Suga, H. & Sagawa, K. (1974). Instantaneous Pressure-Volume Relationships and Their Ratio in the Excised, Supported Canine Left Ventricle, *Circulation Research*, vol.35, pp.117-126

Thomaseth, K. & Cobelli, C. (1999). Generalized Sensitivity Function in Physiological System Identification, *Annals of Biomedical Engineering*, vol.27, no.5, pp.607-616

3

Hemodynamics Study Based on Near-Infrared Optical Assessment

Chia-Wei Sun and Ching-Cheng Chuang
National Yang-Ming University,
Taiwan R.O.C.

1. Introduction

Blood, the body fluid responsible for transport materials and waste products, is composed of cells and plasma. More than 99 percent of the cells in blood are erythrocytes, which carry oxygen from and carbon dioxide to the lungs. The cardiovascular system is responsible for proper blood circulation throughout the body, and the ability of oxygen delivery plays an important role for vital sign monitoring, especially for cardiovascular insufficiency assessment for critical patients with heart failure, septic shock, and cerebral ischemia. Currently, the bedside assessment of cardiovascular adequacy often involves invasive hemodynamic monitoring, and is limited to the measurement of vital signs, blood lactate and capillary refill. Recently, noninvasive evaluation of activation-related tissue oxygenation changes has become available with near-infrared spectroscopy (NIRS). Since the NIRS method can evaluate the spatial distribution of tissue oxygenation in real-time, it has been proposed as an effective tool to quantify changes of local oxygenation in muscle tissue. In order to avoid the use of an exogenous tracer, the analysis of the dynamic response to oxy-hemoglobin (HbO_2) and deoxy-hemoglobin (Hb) during a standardized vascular occlusion test has been proposed for characterizing local metabolic rate, i.e., to analyze the concomitant temporal response of NIRS signal with applied vascular occlusion. Also, the tissue oxygen saturation (StO_2) and total hemoglobin (tHb) changes can be assessed by use of NIRS technique as markers of oxygen consumption and cardiovascular reserve with resting and exercising test.

2. Fundamentals of NIRS and diffuse optical method

2.1 Optical properties of biological tissues

Light propagating in a turbid medium like tissue will be scattered and absorbed by the randomly densely distributed heterogeneities (or particles), which may be cells or large molecules. To describe the absorption, we usually define an absorption coefficient μ_a (in cm^{-1}). The absorption in tissues is due to natural chromophores such as the hemo-pigment of hemoglobin, myoglobin, and bilirubin, the cytochrome pigments of the respiratory chain in the mitochondria, and melanin pigment. For scattering, a scattering coefficient μ_s (in cm^{-1}) is defined. The scattering in tissues is due to discontinuities in refractive index on the microscopic level, such as the aqueous-lipid membrane interfaces surrounding and within each cell or the collagen fibrils within the extracellular matrix. For all optical diagnostic techniques aiming at the identification of pathologic areas, knowledge of the optical properties of tissues is of basic importance for a proper choice of the operation wavelengths. Such a wavelength should maximize the difference between the lesion to be detected and the surrounding healthy tissues, or more generally between the chromophore of interest and any other endogenous or exogenous chromophores present in tissues. The behavior of μ_a as a function of wavelength shows the typical spectral features of the main tissue constituents: blood hemoglobin, lipids, and water (Fig. 1).

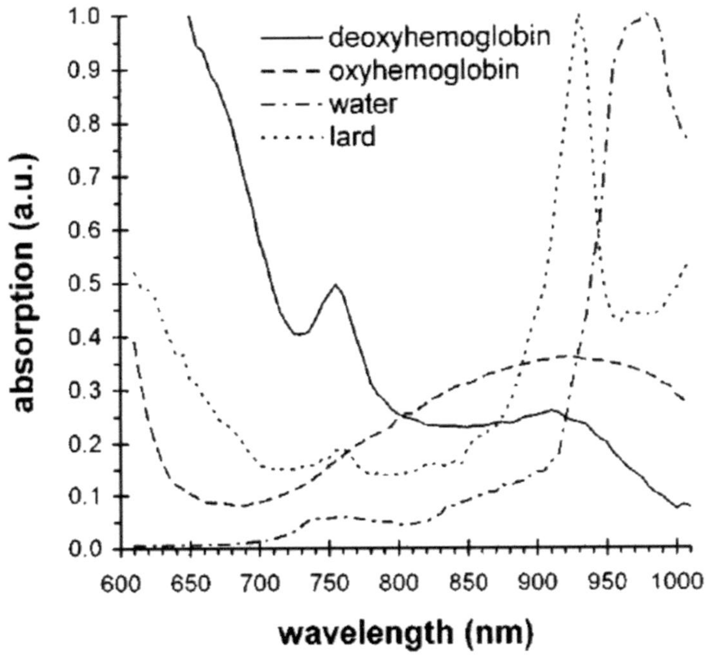

Fig. 1. Absorption spectra of the main tissue constituents: deoxy-hemoglobin (solid curve), oxyhemoglobin (dashed curve), water (dotted curve), and lard (dashed-dotted curve) [Cubeddu et al., 1999].

The transmitted photons can be divided into three types: ballistic (or coherent) photons, snake (or quasi-coherent) photons and diffuse (or multiply scattered) photons. Consider a short optical pulse incident upon a biological tissue. Figure 2 shows all the possibilities of photon scattering. We can see that the ballistic photons pass through the sample without any significant scattering. These photons will arrive at the detector earliest. The ballistic photons propagate in the direction of incoming beam, traverse the shortest path, and retain most information of the incident photons. However, the corresponding light intensity decreases quite rapidly with the propagation distance. Besides, some other photons experience certain forward scattering processes and are classified into the category of snake photon. Snake photons are scattered only slightly in the forward direction and transmit after the ballistic photons. Both ballistic and snake photons travel in the incident direction and arrive earlier than the multiple scattered diffuse photons. Those photons that experience many large-angle scattering processes have unpredicted transmitted angles and lose information. Because of the long traveling path, diffuse photons are delayed in transmission. In some situations, a photon may experience many small-angle plus one large-angle scattering processes. Such a photon contributes to the group of backscattered photon. Because of the zero or weak random scattering, the ballistic, snake and backscattered photons carry more information for sample imaging compared with the diffuse photons.

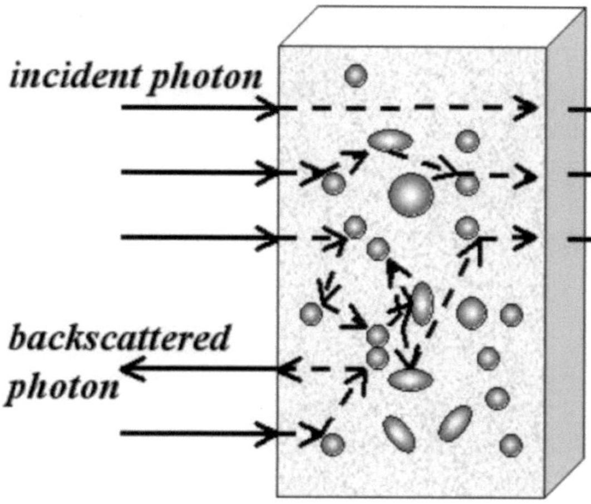

Fig. 2. Illustration of photon migration in a turbid medium.

When light encounters the biological tissue, there will be multiple effects of reflectance, absorption, and scattering due to the inhomogeneity. Even though, each tissue has its own characteristic optical absorption spectra, one can approximate the optical properties of tissues withot that of water, due to the facts of water is the major composition of human body, more than 70%. In blood, there are strong absorption in the visible range due to chromophores such as hemoglobin and bilirubin. Therefore, the absorption is dominated by the blood in tissue. There are also other chromophores that absorb light in the specific spectral range, such as melanin and proteins.

2.2 Light-tissue interaction

Light-tissue interaction, which is the basis for optically probing structure and function at cellular and tissue levels as well for the light-activated photodynamic therapy of cancer and other diseases; benefits from a molecular understanding of cellular and tissue structures and functions. Light propagation in biological tissues is governed by both absorption and scattering processes.

Absorption is the extraction of energy from light by a molecular species. The absorption can be mediated by either a radiative or an irradiative process. Irradiative absorption converts light energy to thermal energy. Radiative absorption introduces flourecence emission of longer wavelengths. Therefore, the ability of light to penetrate tissues depends on how strongly the tissues absorb light. At the short-wavelength end of therapeutic window, the window is bound by the absorption of hemoglobin, in both its oxygenated and deoxygenated forms. The absorption of oxygenated hemoglobin increases approximately two orders of magnitude as the wavelength shortens in the around 600 nm.

Scattering occurs where there is a spatival variation in the refractive index, either continuous or abrupt (e.g., due to localized particles). Scattering events can be further classified into elastic and inelastic ones. In elastic scattering, incident and scattered photons are of the same frequency. Such examples are Mie scattering (e.g., scattering particle size comparable to incident wavelength) and Rayleigh scattering (e.g., scattering particle size is smaller than incident wavelength). In inelastic scattering, incident and scattered photons are of different frequencies. Such examples are Brillouin scattering (e.g., emitting acoustic photons) and Raman scattering (e.g., emitting light of longer wavelengths). The level of inelastic scattering is much weaker as compared with that of elastic scattering, and is therefore negligible in diffuse optical imaging and spectroscopy. In blood, the disk-shaped red cells are the strongest scatters. The erythrocyte disk is ~2 μm thick with a diameter of 7 to 9 μm. The scattering properties of blood are dependent on the hematocrit (volume fraction of red cells) and its degree of agglomeration.

2.3 Near-infrared spectroscopy

NIRS measures tissue absorbance of light at several wavelengths in the spectral region from 600-1000 nm (called therapeutic windows), in which light can penetrate up to several centimeters into biological tissues, enabling deep-tissue imaging and tomography. At shorter wavelengths, the absorption of major tissue chromophores is significantly higher. Conversely, at longer wavelengths, the absorption of water is significantly higher. In addition, absorbing chromophores within biological tissues include such molecular structures as hemoglobin, myoglobin, water, melanin, cytochrome oxidase, bilirubin and

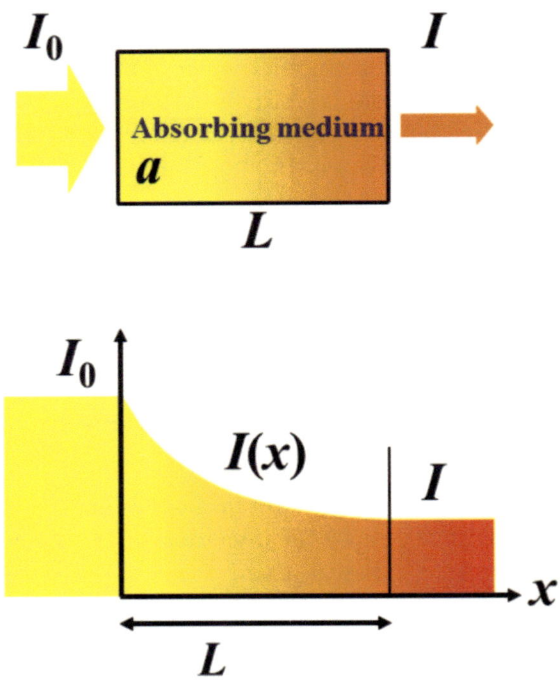

Fig. 3. Diagram of Beer-Lambert absorption of a beam of light as it travels through a slab of width L.

lipids. Contribution of each chromophore to tissue absorption spectrum can be calculated based on their concentrations in different tissue types. Thus enabling determination of concentration changes of oxygenated hemoglobin ([HbO_2]), deoxygenated hemoglobin ([Hb]), blood volume ([HbO_2]+[Hb]) and oxygenated cytochrome-oxidase. Absorption of light by tissue, causing light attenuation, depends on certain compounds that mentioned above. Light attenuation is measured in optical density (*OD*) and can be quantified using the Beer-Lambert's law. In other words, the Beer-Lambert's law relates the absorption of light to the properties of the material through which the light is traveling. The law states that there is a logarithmic dependence between the transmission T, of light through a substance and the product of the absorption coefficient of the substance a, and the distance the light travels through the material L (e.g., the path length). This situation is illustrated by Fig. 3.

Assume that particles may be described as having an absorption cross section (i.e., area), σ, perpendicular to the path of light through a solution, such that a photon of light is absorbed if it strikes the particle, and is transmitted if it does not. Define x as an axis parallel to the direction that photons of light are moving, and dx as the thickness of the slab which light is passing. We assume that dx is sufficiently small that one particle in the slab cannot obscure another particle in the slab when viewed along the x direction. The concentration of particles in the slab is represented by N' (the number density of absorbers). Expressing the number of photons absorbed by the slab as dI, and the total number of photons incident on the slab as I, the fraction of photons absorbed by the slab is given by

$$dI = -\sigma N' I dx \tag{1}$$

$$\frac{dI}{dx} = -\sigma N' I \tag{2}$$

Note that because there are fewer photons which pass through the slab than are incident on it, dI is actually negative (It is proportional in magnitude to the number of photons absorbed). The solution to this simple differential equation is obtained by integrating both sides to obtain I as a function of x

$$\ln(I) = -\sigma N' x + C \tag{3}$$

The difference of intensity for a slab of real thickness L is I_0 at $x = 0$, and I at $x = L$. Using the previous equation, the difference in intensity can be written as

$$\ln(I) - \ln(I_0) = (-\sigma N' L + C) - (-\sigma N' 0 + C) = -\sigma N' L \tag{4}$$

rearranging and exponentiating yields,

$$T = \frac{I}{I_0} = e^{-\sigma N' L} = e^{-\alpha' L} \tag{5}$$

This implies that the absorption is

$$A' = -\ln(T) = -\sigma N' L = -\alpha' L \tag{6}$$

$$A = OD = -\ln(T) = -\ln(\frac{I}{I_0}) = -\alpha LC \tag{7}$$

where C is the concentration of absorbing species in the material.

When light of a known wavelength is used to transilluminate a solution of a compound of unknown concentration *in vitro,* the absorption coefficient and thickness of solution traversed can be substituted in the Beer-Lambert equation to derive the concentration of the substance. Spectroscopy in this form has been used for many years in colorimetric analysis and, in certain circumstances, similar principles can be applied to biological tissue. Thus, in a biological tissue containing different absorbing compounds, the overall attenuation of the incident light at a given wavelength is calculated from the linear sum of the contributions of each compound. There are different absorbers to be considered for NIRS measurements contributing to total light attenuation such as HbO_2 and Hb. These absorbers show different absorption spectra, allowing spectroscopic separation using light of different wavelengths.

2.4 Diffuse optical tomography

The term diffuse optical tomography (DOT) refers to the optical imaging of biological tissue in the diffusive regime. DOT used the harmless near-infrared light that are advantageous because they are non-invasive, less expensive, nonradiative imaging, real-time measurement, compact implementation, long time monitoring, easy operation and the diffuse photon of NIR has a 1/e penetration depth on the order of 0.5 cm, near-infrared in the spectral window of 600-1000 nm wavelength can penetrate several centimeters into human breast tissue. Thus, far DOT has generated a lot of scientific interest and has been applied in various deep-tissue applications such as imaging of brain, breast, limb and joint. According to the type of operation, DOT can be classified into three modes as time domain, frequency domain and continuous wave (Fig. 4).

In all three modes, the reemitted light has the same general form as the source light since the system is linear and time-invariant. In the time domain operation, the optical properties of the tissue are inferred from the temporal point spread function (TPSF), i.e., the temporal response to an ultra-short pulse of light source. Thus, time domain DOT is a kind of "time gating" approach to increase the spatial resolution and it reveals rich depth information. The ballistic photons take the shortest path through the medium, arriving at the detector first. Then, strongly scattered photons (diffused light), arriving with increasing delay, presents a corresponding increase in light path length and transverse excursion uncertainty. In the frequency-domain mode, the source light intensity is amplitude-modulated sinusoidally at typically hundreds of MHz, and the reemitted light modulation has reduced modulation depth (AC amplitude/DC). In the DC mode, the source light is usually time-invariant, but it is sometimes modulated at low frequency (e.g., kHz) to improve the signal-to-noise ratio (SNR) or to encode the source. Such low-frequency modulation, however, does not attain the benefits of the frequency-domain mode. The time-domain and the frequency-domain modes are mathematically related via the Fourier transformation. If measured at many frequencies (including DC) in a sufficiently broad bandwidth, frequency-domain signals can be converted to the time domain using the inverse Fourier transformation. Therefore, the time-domain mode is mathematically equivalent to the combination of the frequency-domain and DC modes. Further, the DC mode is a zero-frequency special case of the frequency-domain mode.

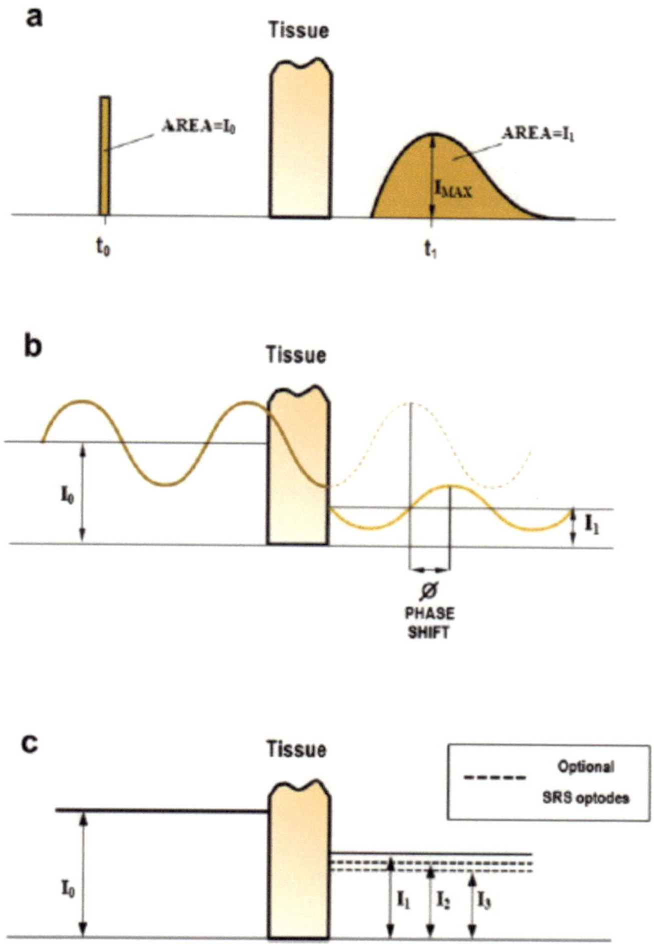

Fig. 4. Source excitation and signal detection for three types of diffuse optical systems. (a) Time domain, (b) Frequency domain, (c) Continuous wave [Pellicer et al., 2011].

DOT offers the capability to simultaneously quantify the tissue concentration of both HbO_2 and Hb. All DOT instrumentation should be designed with the following parameters:

- large dynamic range
- linearity
- stray light rejection
- crosstalk reduction
- long-term stability
- good temporal response

In a DOT system, sources and detectors are placed around the object to be imaged in various geometric configurations. Common geometric configurations, suited for different applications, fall into planar transmission, planar reflection, and cylindrical reemission. Most anatomical sites can be imaged in the planar reflection configuration. Generally, while one source illuminates the object, all detectors measure the reemitted light. This process is repeated with each source to complete a measurement data set; subsequently, images are reconstructed by computer.

3. Monitoring of oxygen consumption and hemodynamic

Local blood flow (BF), expressed in *ml* of blood per 100 ml of tissue per minute, and oxygen consumption (OC), expressed in μmol of O_2 per 100 ml of tissue per minute, are relevant physiological parameters. Over the past decade, NIRS has been shown to be an effective tool for measuring local changes in tissue oxygenation and perfusion. NIRS measures tissue blood flow using different protocols such as the arterial occlusion test (AOT) and the venous occlusion test (VOT). These protocols are noninvasive and allow simultaneous measurements of local BF and OC in skeletal muscles. This technique has demonstrated a strong correlation with xenon and plethysmographic methods, both in resting and exercising subjects. *In situ* muscle oxygen consumption can be measured by NIRS during AOT (the pneumatic cuff is inflated to a pressure of about 240 mm Hg). The increase in Hb during AOT can be attributed to the conversion of HbO_2 into Hb. Although inducing ischemia through arterial occlusion provides additional information on local muscular metabolic energy, this process runs the risk of tissue necrosis in critical patients. Thus, a VOT (the pneumatic cuff is inflated to a pressure of about 50 mm Hg) was adopted to estimate the consumption of oxygen by muscles and blood flow using the same techniques of conventional venous plethysmography. Venous occlusion testing was performed using a controllable pneumatic tourniquet around the upper arm, causing an increase in the volume of blood in the forearm due to undisturbed forearm arterial inflow and interrupted venous outflow. Thus, changes in HbO_2, Hb, and total Hb (tHb) during venous occlusion were induced only through arterial inflow and the consumption of oxygen by tissue. The fundamental measurement associated with the DOSI system is the intensity of light after traveling through the tissue. The intensity of the light signals was measured and analyzed according to the modified Beer-Lambert law. The modified Beer-Lambert law is as follows:

$$OD = -\log(\frac{I}{I_0}) = \varepsilon CLB + G \tag{8}$$

where OD is the optical density. I_0 and I are the intensity of incident light and detected light, respectively. ε represents the extinction coefficient of the tissue; C is the concentration of the tissue. L represents the mean path length of detected photons. B is the path length factor set for the compensation of various effective path lengths of various wavelengths. G is defined as the geometric factor used to compensate the objective with different geometrical shapes. Typically, L, B and G are constants with monochromatic illumination in a turbid media with unchanging geometry. Changes in optical signaling were measured concomitantly with changes in the oxygenation of tissue. Then equation (8) can be rewritten as:

$$\Delta OD = OD_{Final} - OD_{Initial} = -\log(\frac{I_f}{I_i}) = \varepsilon \Delta CLB \tag{9}$$

where ΔOD is the change in optical density. OD_{Final} and $OD_{Initial}$ are detected optical density and the optical density of incident light. If and I_i are the measured intensities before and after the change in concentration; ΔC is the change in concentration. Changes in detected light intensity were dominated by changes in the concentration of HbO_2 and Hb in the tissue. Therefore, the description can be treated as follows:

$$\Delta OD^{\lambda} = (\varepsilon_{HbO_2}^{\lambda} \cdot \Delta[HbO_2] + \varepsilon_{Hb}^{\lambda} \cdot \Delta[Hb])B^{\lambda}L \tag{10}$$

$$\Delta[HbO_2] = \frac{\varepsilon_{Hb}^{\lambda_1} \cdot (\Delta OD^{\lambda_2} / B^{\lambda_2}) - \varepsilon_{Hb}^{\lambda_2} \cdot (\Delta OD^{\lambda_1} / B^{\lambda_1})}{(\varepsilon_{Hb}^{\lambda_1} \cdot \varepsilon_{HbO_2}^{\lambda_2} - \varepsilon_{Hb}^{\lambda_2} \cdot \varepsilon_{HbO_2}^{\lambda_1})L} \tag{11}$$

$$\Delta[Hb] = \frac{\varepsilon_{HbO_2}^{\lambda_2} \cdot (\Delta OD^{\lambda_1} / B^{\lambda_1}) - \varepsilon_{HbO_2}^{\lambda_1} \cdot (\Delta OD^{\lambda_2} / B^{\lambda_2})}{(\varepsilon_{Hb}^{\lambda_1} \cdot \varepsilon_{HbO_2}^{\lambda_2} - \varepsilon_{Hb}^{\lambda_2} \cdot \varepsilon_{HbO_2}^{\lambda_1})L} \tag{12}$$

$$B = \frac{1}{2}\sqrt{\frac{3\mu_s^{'}}{\mu_a}}\left[1 - \frac{1}{(1 + L\sqrt{3\mu_s^{'}\mu_a})}\right] \tag{13}$$

The oxygenation saturation StO_2 and the concentration of total hemoglobin can be calculated from concentrations of HbO_2 and Hb based on Eqs. (14) and (15):

$$StO_2 = \frac{\Delta[HbO_2]}{\Delta[HbO_2] + \Delta[Hb]} \tag{14}$$

$$tHb = \Delta[HbO_2] + \Delta[Hb] \tag{15}$$

Generally, temporally-applied low cuff pressures (50 mm Hg in our cases) occlude venous outflow while minimizing the obstruction of arterial inflow. An increase in deoxygenated

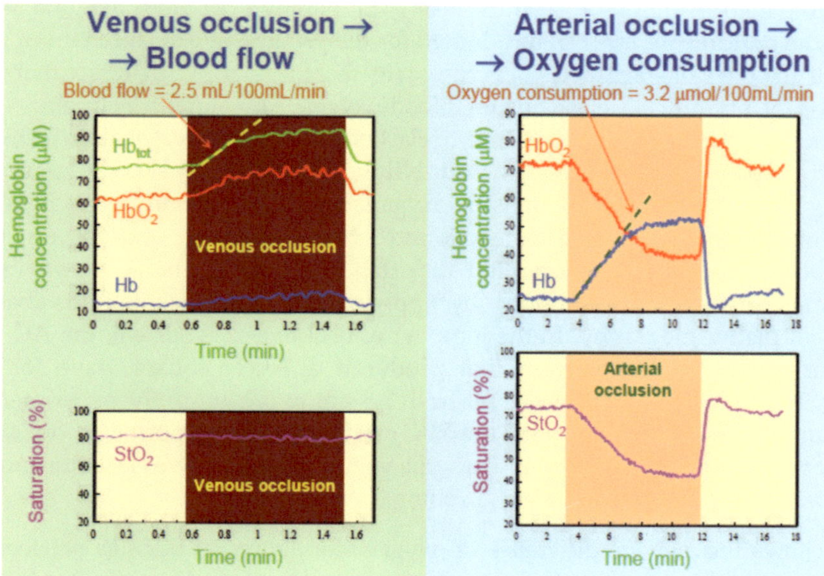

Fig. 5. Changes in forearm hemoglobin concentration and saturation induced by VOT (left) and AOT (right) in the upper arm [Sergio Fantini's Group, Department of Biomedical Engineering, Tufts University].

blood is then used to determine the level of oxygenation in muscle. Near-infrared spectroscopy assesses the level of oxygenation and the volume of blood in local tissue, and VOT has been shown to provide results in agreement with those obtained from traditional measurements employing plethysmography with calculations based on the Fick principle.

Figure 5 shows typical traces of hemoglobin concentration and saturation measured in the brachioradialis muscle (forearm) of a human subject during VOT and AOT. The main effect of the venous occlusion is to increase the hemoglobin concentration, as a result of blood accumulation. The tissue desaturation during arterial occlusion results from a rate of decrease of [HbO_2] that is equal to the rate of increase of [Hb] because the [tHb] remains constant during arterial occlusion. The initial rate of increase of [tHb] during VOT can be translated into a measurement of BF. The initial rate of increase of [Hb] during AOT can be translated into a measurement of the oxygen consumption.

4. The correlation between tissue oxygenation and erythrocytes elasticity

The change of tissue oxygenation resulted from several physiological conditions: cardiac output, pulmonary circulation, systemic circulation, oxygen consumption of tissue, and characterization of red blood cells (RBCs). Human erythrocytes have the shape of a biconcave disk (approximately 7 μm in diameter), which imparts a high surface-to-volume ratio so that oxygen and carbon dioxide can rapidly diffuse to and from the interior of the cell. Erythrocytes are highly deformable, which is essential for them to pass through small capillaries in microcirculation circuits. Furthermore, the deformability reveals the inherent property of erythrocytes that has been proved for differentiation between normal RBCs and malaria-infected RBCs. In this case, malaria-infected RBCs are manifested to be much less deformable, in comparison with normal RBCs. Optical tweezers have been utilized to quantify the deformability of erythrocytes with noninvasive trapping and stretching. Although the optical tweezers can be adopted for the probing of RBC mechanical properties that reveals the physiological states of erythrocyte, there is no direct evidence that shows the contribution of erythrocyte elasticity for blood-oxygen supplement in human circulation system. The correlation between erythrocyte elasticity and tissue oxygenation is investigated based on jumping optical tweezers and NIRS measurement. When the noninvasive monitoring the dynamic response to tissue oxygenation during an induced ischemia process by AOT could characterize local metabolic rate of muscle energy and tissue oxygenation recovery behavior with the assumption that tHb is constant. The AOT was utilized to estimate muscle oxygen consumption by applying the same technique as that used in conventional plethysmography. In the jumping optical tweezers system, the AC voltage is used to drive the diffracted beam that produced a 1-kHz square wave for the RBC stretching. The jumping distances are set from 3.8 μm to 5.9 μm in the experiments. In the Kelvin–Voigt viscoelastic solid model, the RBC can be treated as a spring model with elastic constant k and damping coefficient b. Thus, the values of erythrocyte elasticity and viscosity can be obtained from jumping tweezers probing.

Figure 6. shows the average difference of oxygenation temporal tracings between the two groups. Generally, both temporal profiles demonstrate the typical pattern that indicates the isolated increase in metabolic rate of oxygen based on a one-compartment model. The Hb rising is caused by oxygen consumption by arterial occlusion followed reactive hyperemia. The concentration of HbO_2 declines under the concomitant condition of oxygen supplement

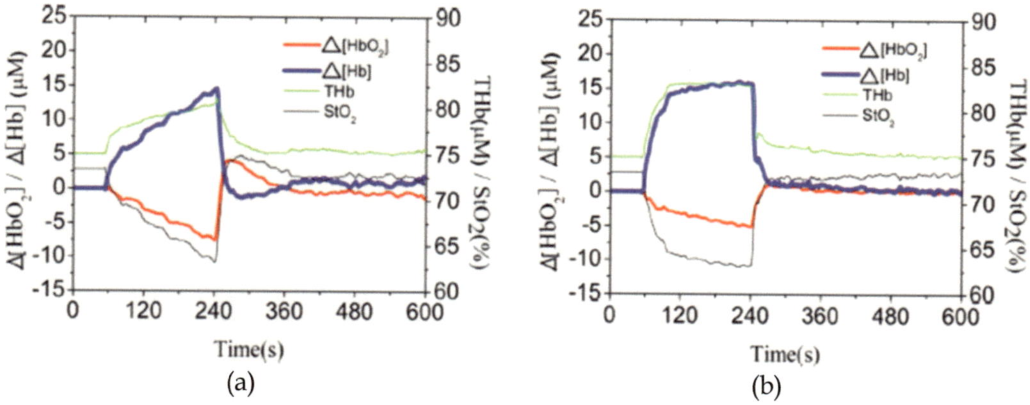

Fig. 6. Temporal tracings of tissue oxygen saturation (StO_2), total hemoglobin (THb), oxy-hemoglobin (HbO_2) and deoxy-hemoglobin (Hb) response to an AOT assessment: (a) the slower response of oxygenation dynamics, and (b) the faster response of oxygenation dynamics [Wu et al., 2011].

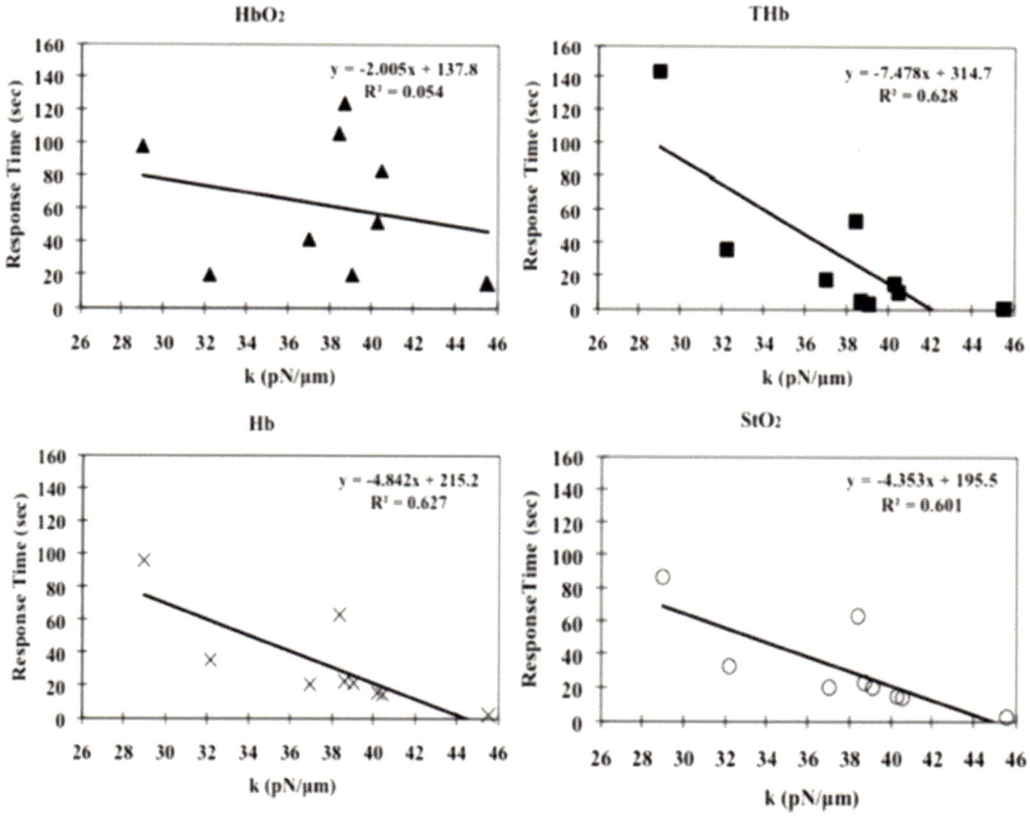

Fig. 7. The correlation between the response time of oxygenation signal and erythrocyte elasticity. The R^2 values for elastic constant versus response time of HbO_2, Hb, tHb and (d) StO_2 [Wu et al., 2011].

interrupted to the muscle. Group 1 is a slower change rate of oxygenation during AOT. Quantitatively, the increasing time of Hb concentration to 80% of the maximum value is more than 100 s in group 1. On the contrary, the dynamic oxygenation signals of AOT from group 2 respond faster than group 1.

The interpretation of the results from NIRS and optical tweezers is based on an assumption: the AOT-induced dynamic oxygenation signal is dependent on the related erythrocytes elasticity in vessels. The lower k implies higher deformability of RBC. During the application of high pressure on the extremity, the vessels were blocked for blood circulation. RBC with higher deformability may offer more oxygen supplement to muscle because of its higher passing ability in obstructed vessels. This phenomenon can be indicated from the tardier rising/falling of oxygenation tracings during AOT in group 1. The correlations are linearly fitted between the erythrocyte elastic constant and the response time of HbO_2, Hb, tHb, and StO_2 in Fig. 7. The response time is defined as the time spent while the oxygenation response reached the half-maximum value after arterial occlusion. The coefficient of determination R^2 (the square of the correlation coefficient) is than calculated for each case. Thus, the RBC elasticity is more strongly related to the Hb response than HbO_2, e.g. the change of Hb concentration dominates the correlation between erythrocyte elasticity and AOT-induced tissue oxygenation dynamics. Besides, similar evidence is also revealed in tHb and StO_2 plots. This result is reasonable because the tHb and StO_2 signals are both led from changes of Hb. The experimental results show a linear correlation between the oxygenation signal caused by AOT and the elasticity of erythrocytes.

5. The clinical applications of the near-infrared oxygenation monitoring

5.1 Cerebral oxygenation

The high sensitivity of NIRS to changes in the tissue hemoglobin concentration (changes as small as 0.05-0.10 μM in tissues can be detected) affords the optical detection of small cerebral hemodynamic fluctuations. NIRS is a promising non-invasive brain imaging technique with a high sampling rate, precise and localized spatial resolution. The NIRS technique provides information about the slow signal (i.e., hemoglobin response) and fast signal (i.e., neuronal activation) of neuron-vascular coupling (Fig. 8). The slow signal occurs in the range of seconds after the onset of the stimulation and reflects mainly changes in light absorption property in brain. On the contrary, the fast signal is believed to result from light scatter changes that are associated with ion currents across the neural membrane, which appear in the range of milliseconds after stimulation.

Neurovascular coupling is the generic term for changes in cerebral metabolic rate of oxygen ($CMRO_2$), cerebral blood flow (CBF), and cerebral blood volume (CBV) related to brain activity. NIRS detects changes in [HbO_2] and [Hb] and therefore total hemoglobin concentration [tHb], which corresponds to CBV. CBF and $CMRO_2$ also affect the [HbO_2] and [Hb] traces. Assuming a one-compartment model (Fig. 9), an isolated change in CBF will have the depicted effect on the [HbO_2] and [Hb]. The increase in CBF will lead to an increase in [HbO_2] and a decrease in [Hb] because more oxygenated than deoxygenated blood will fill the compartment. This effect is often described as the washout effect. Note that the changes are completely symmetrical. This NIRS method permitted several benefits as non-invasive, less expensive, non-ionizing radiation imaging, real-time measurement, compact implementation, long time monitoring and easy operation with high time resolution and

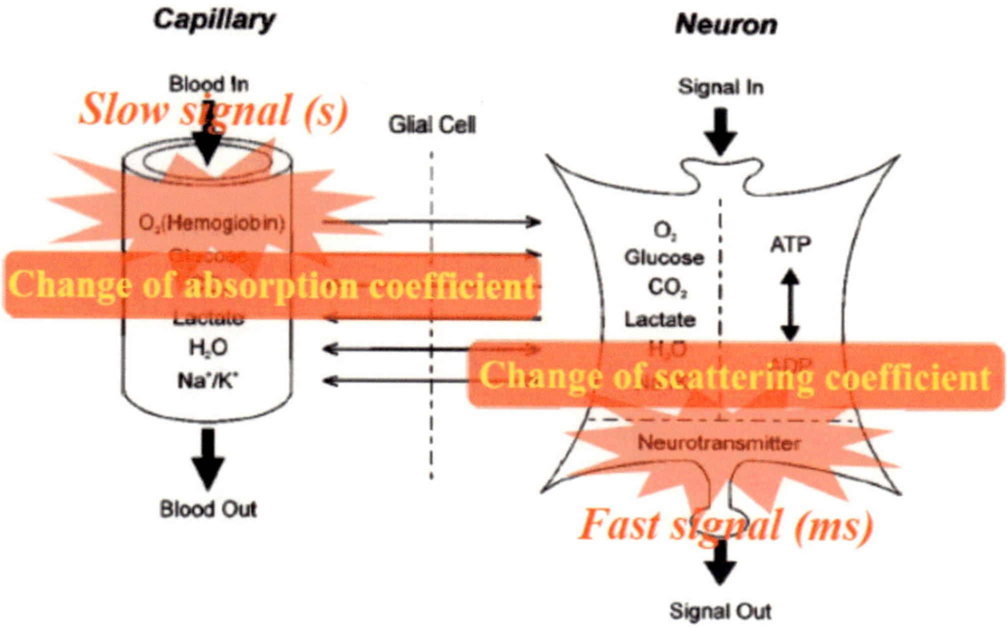

Fig. 8. Neuron-vascular coupling

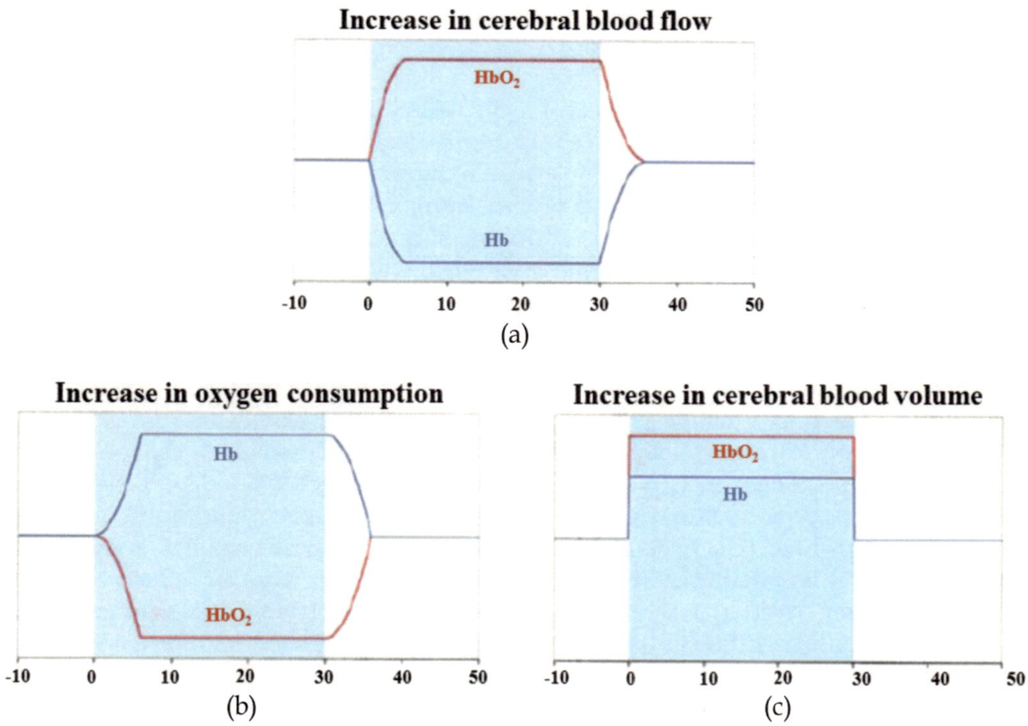

Fig. 9. The effect of an isolated increase in cerebral blood flow (a), cerebral metabolic rate of oxygen (b), or total hemoglobin concentration (c) on the time evolution of the [HbO_2] and [Hb] as predicted by the one-compartment model [Wolf et al., 2001].

adequate spatial resolution for continuously recording [HbO_2] and [Hb] changes of brain. Also, NIRS offers a more comprehensive measurement of brain activity than blood-oxygenation-level-dependent (BOLD) functional magnetic resonance imaging (fMRI).

Thus, NIRS can be used as a continuous monitor of changes in cerebral oxygenation and blood volume by following changes in the concentrations of [HbO_2] and [Hb]. It is also possible to make absolute measurements of CBF and CBV. NIRS has been applied to the measurement of tissue blood flow by using a small change in [HbO_2] as a tracer and applying a modification of the Fick principle which states that the amount of substance taken up by an organ per unit time is equivalent to the difference between the rate of the arrival of the substance, calculated as the product of blood flow through the organ by the arterial concentration of the substance, and the rate of the departure of the substance from the organ, calculated as the venous concentration of the substance. A small reduction in arterial saturation (of the order of 5%) is induced by lowering fractional inspired oxygen FiO_2. When a stable baseline is achieved, a breath of 100% oxygen creates a bolus of [HbO_2] in the arterial circulation which acts as the required Fick tracer. The rate of arrival of [HbO_2] in the brain a few seconds later can be observed by NIRS. CBF may be calculated by considering the ratio of the rate of tracer accumulation in the organ to the amount of tracer delivered. The accumulation of [HbO_2] in the brain is dependent on both arterial inflow and venous outflow.

The signal representing the difference between the change in [HbO_2] and [Hb] concentration, termed Δ HbD, is twice the amplitude of the signal corresponding to [HbO_2] change in concentration alone, therefore

$$CBF(ml.100^{-1}.min^{-1}) = k_1 \cdot (\Delta\ HbD)/2 \cdot H \cdot \int 0 \rightarrow t \cdot \Delta\ SaO_2 \quad (16)$$

where K_1 is a constant reflecting the molecular weight of hemoglobin and cerebral tissue density; $\Delta\ SaO_2$ is the change in arterial oxygen saturation by pulse oximetry; and H is the blood vessel hemoglobin concentration (g/dL). Application of this technique in the clinical field was demonstrated by Edwards and colleagues who showed that i.v. indomethacin administered to close a patent ductus arteriosus led to a marked decrease in CBF measured by NIRS.

Notwithstanding that CBF is the hemodynamic variable most familiar to clinicians, a combination of this information with other variables such as CBV would be valuable in interpreting changes in the clinical condition. Continuous measurement of changes in [tHb] generally reflects changes in CBV. Absolute quantification of CBV is also possible with NIRS. If arterial saturation is reduced by a small increment (approximately 5%) in a slow and controlled manner [HbO_2] is observed by NIRS to decline in parallel. As with CBF measurement, it is important that the change is small enough to avoid any effects on CBF or oxygen extraction. If arterial saturation is plotted against [HbO_2], the gradient of the resulting straight line is directly proportional to CBV. CBV can be calculated in absolute terms using a modification of a standard indicator dilution principle. Absolute CBV value can be derived from:

$$CBV(ml.100g^{-1}) = k_2 \cdot (\Delta\ HbD)/2 \cdot H \cdot \Delta\ SaO_2 \quad (17)$$

where K_2 is obtained from K_1 and the large-vessel: tissue hematocrit ratio.

Consider a brain empty of blood. However much arterial saturation was varied, there could be no change in cerebral HbO_2 concentration and the gradient of the line would be zero. In contrast, a head with a high CBV would display a large change in [HbO_2] for a small change in arterial saturation. As the units of the gradient are unfamiliar in the raw state it must be converted to CBV in the same way as described for tHb. This measurement can be used to provide a baseline value for CBV with which the real-time trends in [tHb] can be compared. Changes in cerebral intravascular oxygenation, equivalent to the difference between [HbO_2] and [Hb], are an indicator of the mean oxygensaturation of hemoglobin in all types of blood vessels (arteries, capillaries and veins) in tissue. Thus, changes in cerebral blood volume can be assessed from changes in Δ [tHb], CBV can calculate by the proportionalities:

$$\Delta\ CBV=k_2 \times \Delta\ [tHb]/H \tag{18}$$

5.2 Near-infrared spectroscopy and imaging for breast cancer

NIRS has been used for clinical detection of various cancers, such as breast cancer, skin cancer, bladder cancer, lung cancer, brain tumors, and cervical cancer. For human breast imaging, NIRS reveals pathological tumor contrast directly in vascularity, hemoglobin concentration and tissue scattering property. Based on the modified Beer-Lambert's Law, the change of vascularity and oxygenation can be observed by utilizing optical measurements at multiple source-detector positions on the tissue surfaces. NIRS techniques use measurements of transmitted light to produce spatially resolved images. Images of the absorption or scattering properties of the tissue, or other physiological parameters such as tHb and StO_2 may be generated. Because the low spatial resolution in NIRS imaging technique, at present, the new diagnostic methods of NIRS imaging focusing on physiological properties detected of the breast tumor such as the hemoglobin response. In the case of human breast tissue, functional activation is not available and instead spatial differences must be employed. Localization and characterization of the incremental changes of optical properties with respect to position changes are necessary. Thus, the problem is significant and absolute values of optical properties involve problems of the physiological and biochemical baselines for distinguishing pathologies from normal and tumor region. The overall average tHb concentration and StO_2 for benign fibroadenoma and malignant lesions suggest that breast lesions contain at least twice the tHb concentration of healthy background breast tissue. This is supported by evidence suggesting that breast lesions have greater tHb concentrations compares to background tissues.

Some study provided specificity and sensitivity values to describe the ability of near-infrared imaging to detect malignancy based on spectroscopic information. One of study performed by Chance et al. was a 6 year, two site experiments that involved the use of a multi-wavelength handheld device, operating in CW domain. Data was acquired from 166 patients of whom 44 patients had confirmed malignancy and the remainder classified as non-cancer patients. Blood volume and saturations were calculated with reference to a similar location on the contralateral healthy breast. The results are summarized in the 2D normogram of blood volume and oxygen saturation in Fig. 10. The abscissa is relative increments of blood concentration in units of micro-molar concentration change with respect to the average cancer-free value. The ordinate represents incremental change with respect to the average cancer-free value in percent change of hemoglobin saturation. In this graph, verified cancers are indicated with a dot and cancer-free breasts plotted with an X. The normogram can be divided into two zones, one containing the verified cancers (I) and the other containing cancer-free breasts (II). This technique was able to distinguish cancer from non-cancer bearing breasts with 96% sensitivity and 93% specificity, with an area under the curve of 95%.

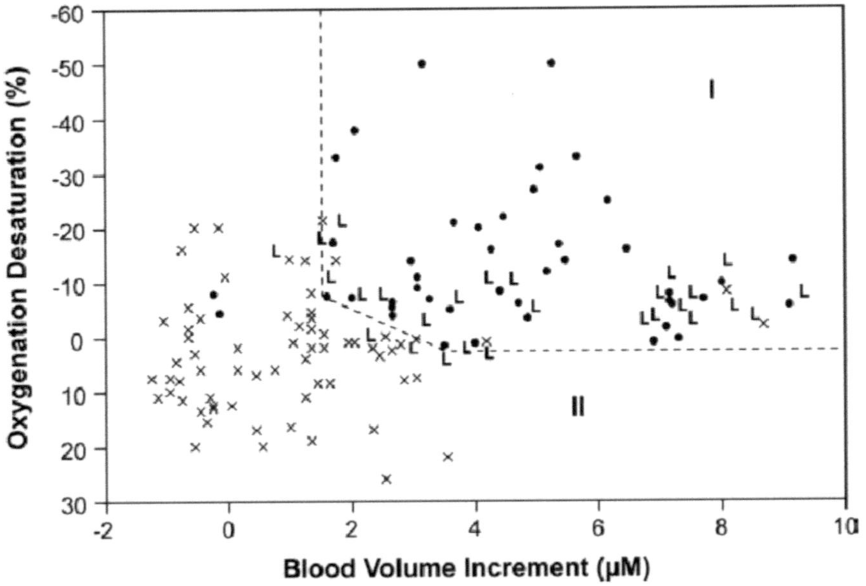

Fig. 10. A two-dimensional nomogram display of currently available NIR breast cancer data [Chance et al., 2005].

5.3 Intensive care unit

In intensive care medicine, real-time physiological monitoring of vital signs plays an important role in diagnosis and therapy, particularly for the cardiovascular assessment of patients with heart failure and/or sepsis. To maintain central blood pressure and vital organ perfusion, cardiovascular insufficiency may be overcome by increasing sympathetic output through the vasoconstriction of lesser vital organs and muscles. Unfortunately, this compensatory mechanism often masks profound hypovolemia. Currently, bedside assessment of cardiovascular adequacy involves either the measurement of the vital signs, blood lactate levels, and capillary refill, or the monitoring of tissue oxygenation using invasive techniques. The ability to characterize tissue oxygenation through non-invasive means would be of immense benefit in the intensive care unit (ICU). The approach of NIRS also can highly valuable for examining the effects of medication in the ICU.

Figure 11 (a) shows the group average response with a standard deviation of tHb and StO_2 for the VOT of normal subjects, respectively. Figure 11 (b) shows the tHb and StO_2 curves in response to the VOT in patients with heart failure. Obviously, the average response of tHb for patients with heart failure is lower and more slurred than that of normal subjects. A stepwise decreasing pattern in patients with heart failure characterized StO_2 tracing.

The NIRS is capable of accessing the spatial distribution of tissue oxygenation, and to do so in real-time. For qualitative comparisons, the greatest change in tissue oxygenation occurred at the beginning of VOT in healthy subjects, particularly with regard to changes in the concentration of oxy-hemoglobin. Different temporal tracings reveal different physiological conditions. The temporal tracings of tissue oxygenation are measured using NIRS measurement and a VOT, employing normal subjects and ICU patients suffering from heart failure. The NIRS provides a highly potential on the oxygenation of muscles in the extremities measured during VOT in normal subjects and ICU patients.

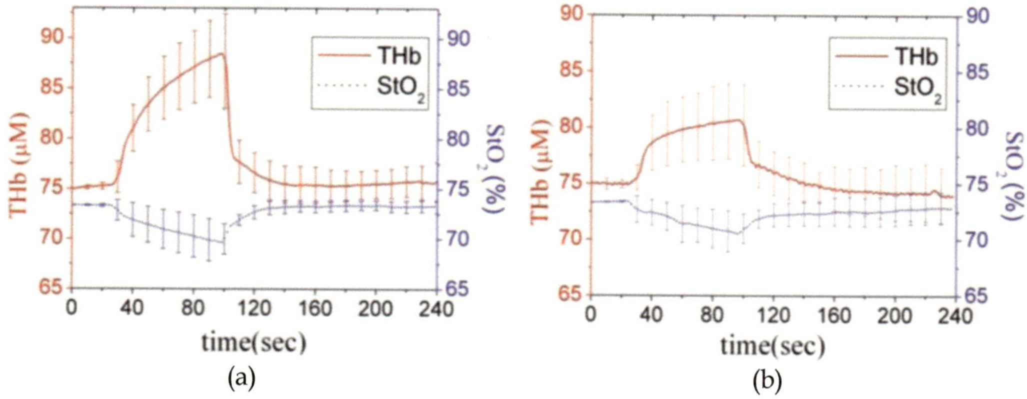

Fig. 11. Temporal tracings of the VOT response from normal control and heart failure patient tissue oxygen saturation (StO_2) and total hemoglobin (tHb) response [Wang et al., 2011].

5.4 The exercising test

NIRS is applied to study tissue oxygenation in skeletal muscle and brain under a variety of experimental conditions. The local hemoglobin status and blood flow is an important parameter for assessment of muscle physiology, particularly during exercise in both healthy and disease. The optical measurement of the near-infrared absorption coefficient at multiple wavelengths can be translated into measurements of the [HbO_2] and [Hb] in tissue. During exercise, both blood flow and oxidative metabolism in skeletal muscle respond to meet increased oxygen demand.

Figure 12 reports the results of an experiment to measure the desaturation in the legs of peripheral vascular disease (PVD) patients during stationary bicycle exercise. The comparison of the typical hemoglobin saturation traces recorded on healthy subject (blue line) and PVD patient (red line) in Fig. 12 shows the difference in the response of healthy and diseased legs. In the healthy subject, the hemoglobin saturation decreases slightly during the exercise, whereas the PVD patient shows a consistent decrease in hemoglobin saturation. The recovery time after exercise is also significantly shorter in the healthy subject than in the PVD patient. These results are consistent with an insufficient blood flow adjustment in the PVD patients to compensate for the increased oxygen demands during muscle exercise. The longer recovery time is also associated with the lower blood flow so that it requires more time to overcome the oxygen debt. In addition, the ability to characterize the muscular performance of athletes, during and after exercise leads to vital information in the field of sports medicine. These measurements may monitor the muscle tissue oxygenation and hemodynamics and assist in determining an athlete's exercise capacity, assessing the efficacy and validity of training programs and tracking an athlete's progress while in rehabilitative conditioning.

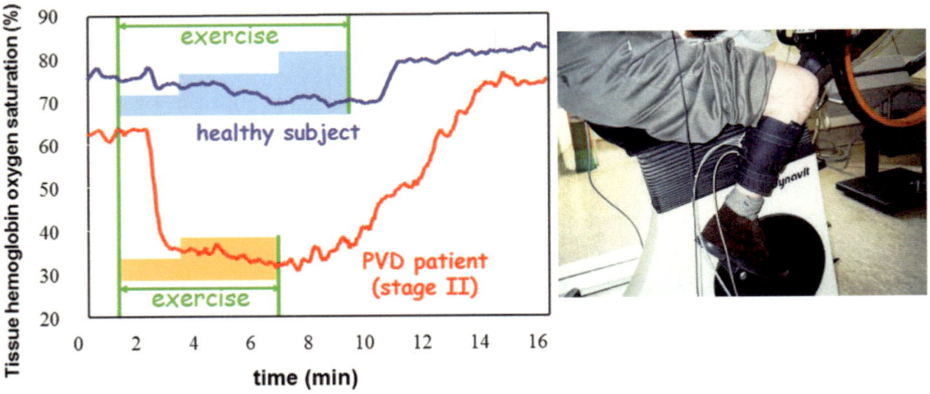

Fig. 12. Typical hemoglobin saturation traces of healthy and PVD patient [Sergio Fantini's Group, Department of Biomedical Engineering, Tufts University and in collaboration with R. Palumbo and G. Vaudo, Policlinico Monteluce, University of Perugia, Italy].

Knowledge of how the central nervous system (CNS) influences motor neurons to limit neuromuscular performance is nascent. It is accepted that motor command and its corollaries exist at multiple levels in the CNS to sustain homeostatic functions during exercise. Likewise, several metabolic and neurochemical pathways between skeletal

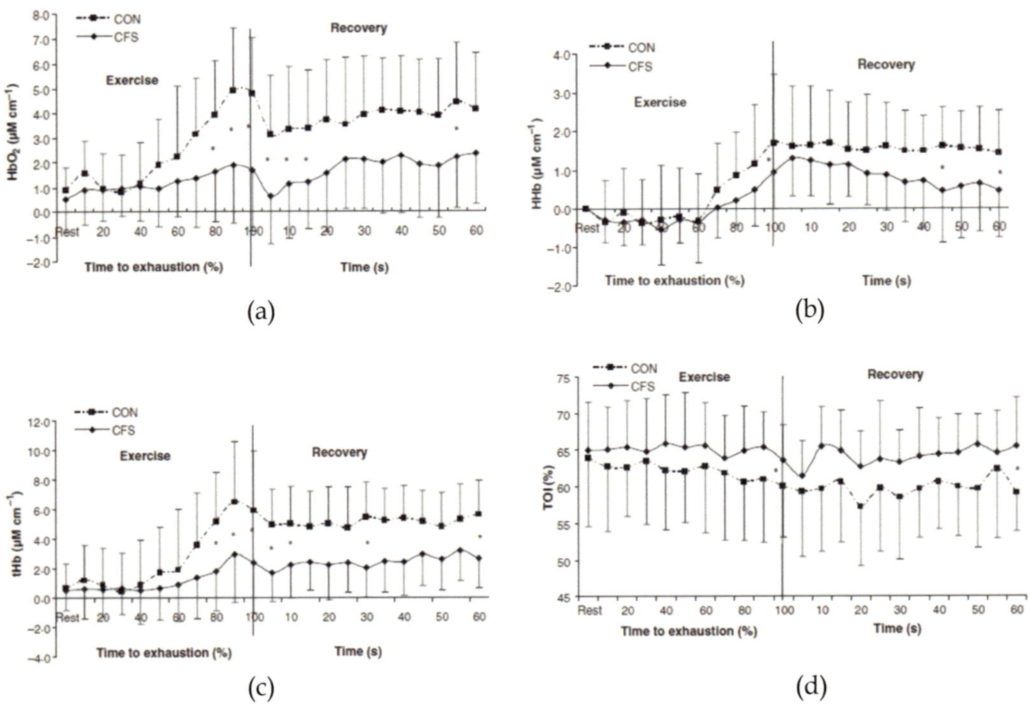

Fig. 13. Left prefrontal cortex (a) oxy-haemoglobin changes (HbO_2; lM cm); (b) deoxy-haemoglobin changes (HHb; lM cm); (c) total blood volume changes (tHb; lM cm) and (d) tissue oxygenation index (TOI %) in the chronic fatigue syndrome (CFS) and control (CON) subjects during continuous incremental maximal exercise and resting recovery [Neary et al., 2008].

muscles, the spinal cord, and the brain suggest ways by which exercise might influence the CNS. The studies of the brain during exercise have focused on cerebral hemodynamic responses. The use of NIRS to evaluate hemodynamic changes in the brain during exercise has increased as NIRS systems have become more available.

Figure 13 demonstrates the effects of maximal incremental exercise (performed an incremental cycle ergometer test to exhaustion) on cerebral oxygenation in chronic fatigue syndrome (CFS) and control (CON) subjects. Prefrontal cortex HbO_2, Hb and tHb were significantly lower at maximal exercise in CFS versus CON, as was TOI during exercise and recovery. The CFS subjects exhibited significant exercise intolerance and reduced prefrontal oxygenation and tHb response when compared with CON subjects. These data suggest that the altered cerebral oxygenation and blood volume may contribute to the reduced exercise load in CFS, and supports the contention that CFS, in part, is mediated centrally.

NIRS has been used as a practical indicator of cerebral oxygenation and hemodynamic change during sub-maximal and maximal exercise. As NIRS technology continues to improve, considerations of optode distance and location, and reconsideration of and use of quantifiable light signals will expand the information that can be obtained using NIRS during and after exercise to understand cortical brain function and its role in human performance and health, especially when NIRS is used with other neuroimaging measures concurrent with controlled manipulations of the brain.

5.5 Hemodialysis patients

Hemodialysis has direct and indirect effects on skin and muscle microcirculatory regulation that are severe enough to worsen tolerance to physical exercise and muscle asthenia in patients undergoing dialysis. Hemodialysis utilizes counter current flow, where the dialysate is flowing in the opposite direction to blood flow in the extracorporeal circuit. Several side effects, including low blood pressure, fatigue, chest pains, nausea, headaches and muscle-cramps, are originated by removing too much fluid rapidly. The patients on long-term hemodialysis suffer from a variety of syndrome problems, for example, muscle-cramps (ex: shoulder pain). Meanwhile, it leads to reduce oxygen concentration, especially with the ipsilateral of the arteriovenous fistula. NIRS has been shown to be an effective tool for measuring local changes of tissue in hemodynamics.

Diffuse optical imaging and spectroscopy with near-infrared light reconstructs tissue physiologic parameters based on noninvasive measurement of tissue optical properties. NIRS can provide a high potential to be extensively employed to evaluate human hemodynamics, and to widely use and explain in several clinical applications. The advantages brought by NIRS compared with the conventional techniques are numerous: it allows a non-invasive, real-time measurement of the concentrations of interest, the observation time is unlimited, it can be used to monitor the time evolution of the tissue oxygenation during physiological or metabolic processes, it uses instrumentation of relatively small dimensions and it is cost effective. All these characteristics are fundamental for clinical use. Furthermore, the optical method can provide completely "patient-oriented" measurement for clinical applications.

6. References

Ahmadi S., Sinclair P. J. and Davis G. M., Muscle oxygenation following concentric exercise, *Isokinet. Exerc. Sci.*, Vol. 15, pp. 309-319, 2007.

Blasi R. A. De, Palmisani S., Alampi D., Mercieri M., Romano R., Collini S. and Pinto G., Microvascular dysfunction and skeletal muscle oxygenation assessed by phase-modulation near-infrared spectroscopy in patients with septic shock, *Intensive Care Med.*, Vol. 31, pp. 1661-1668, 2005.

Beekvelt M. C. P. van, Engelen B. G. M. van, Wevers R. A. and Colier W. N. J. M., In vivo quantitative near-infrared spectroscopy in skeletal muscle during incremental isometric handgrip exercise, *Clin. Physiol. & Func. Im.*, Vol. 22, pp. 210-217, 2002.

Boas D. A., Gaudette T., Strangman G., Cheng X., Marota J. J. A. and Mandeville J. B., The accuracy of near-infrared spectroscopy and imaging during focal changes in cerebral hemodynamics, *NeuroImage*, Vol. 13, pp. 76-90, 2001.

Boushel R., Langberg H., Olesen J., Gonzales-Alonzo J., Bu¨low J. and Kjær M., Monitoring tissue oxygen availability with near infrared spectroscopy (NIRS) in health and disease, *Scand. J. Med. Sci. Sports*, Vol. 11, pp. 213-222, 2001.

Boushel R., Langberg H., Olesen J., Nowak M., Simonsen L., Bülow J. and Kjær M., Regional blood flow during exercise in humans measured by near-infrared spectroscopy and indocyanine green, *J. Appl. Physiol.*, Vol. 89, pp. 1868-1878, 2000.

Beekvelt M. C. P. Van, Colier W. N., Engelen B. G. M. van, Hopman M. T. E., Wevers R. A. and Oeseburg B., Validation of measurement protocols to assess oxygen consumption and blood flow in the human forearm by near infrared spectroscopy, *Proc. SPIE*, Vol. 3194, pp. 133-144, 1998.

Blasi R. A. De, Almenräder N., Aurisicchio P. and Ferrari M., Comparison of two methods of measuring forearm oxygen consumption (VO_2) by near-infrared spectroscopy, *J. Biomed. Opt.*, Vol. 2, pp. 171-175, 1997.

Belardinelli R., Barstow T. J., Porszasz J. and Wasserman K., Changes in skeletal muscle oxygenation during incremental exercise measured with near infrared spectroscopy, *Eur J. Appl. Physiol.*, Vol. 70, pp. 487-492, 1995.

Blasi R. A. De, Ferrari M., Natali A., Conti G., Mega A. and Gasparetto A., Noninvasive measurement of forearm blood flow and oxygen consumption by near-infrared spectroscopy, *J. Appl. Physiol.*, Vol. 76, pp. 1388-1393, 1994.

Chance B., Nioka S., Zhang J., Conant E. F., Hwang E., Briest S., Orel S. G., Schnall M. D. and Czerniecki B. J., Breast cancer detection based on incremental biochemical and physiological properties of breast cancers: A six-year, two-site study[1], *Acad. Radiol.*, Vol. 12, pp. 925-933, 2005.

Casavola C., Paunescu L. A., Fantini S. and Gratton E., Blood flow and oxygen consumption with near-infrared spectroscopy and venous occlusion: spatial maps and the effect of time and pressure of inflation, *J. Bio. Opt.*, Vol. 5, pp. 269-276, 2000.

Cubeddu R., Pifferi A., Taroni P., Torricelli A. and Valentini G., Noninvasive absorption and scattering spectroscopy of bulk diffusive media: An application to the optical characterization of human breast, *Applied Physics Letters*, Vol. 74, pp. 874-876, 1999.

Casavola C., Paunescu L. A., Fantini S., Franceschini M. A., Lugarà P. M. and Gratton E., Application of near-infrared tissue oxymetry to the diagnosis of peripheral vascular disease, *Clin. Hemorheol. Micro.*, Vol. 21, pp. 389-393, 1999.

Chance B., Optical method, *Annu. Rev. Biophys. Biophys. Chern.*, Vol. 20, pp. 1-28, 1991.

Dinh T. V., Biomedical photonics handbook, *Boca Raton London & New York*, 2003.

Edward A. D., Wyatt J. S., Richardson C., Potter A., Reynolds E. O. R., Cope M. and Delpy D. T., Effects of indomethacin on cerebral haemodynamics in very preterm infants, *The Lancet*, Vol. 335, pp. 1491-1495, 1990.

Fantini's S. Group, Optical study of muscle hemodynamics and oxygenation, Department of Biomedical Engineering, Tufts University. http://ase.tufts.edu/biomedical/research/fantini/research.asp

Hachiya T., Blaber A. P. and Saito M., Near-infrared spectroscopy provides an index of blood flow and vasoconstriction in calf skeletal muscle during lower body negative pressure, *Acta. Physiol.*, Vol. 193, pp. 117-127, 2008.

Homma S., Eda H., Ogasawara S. and Kagaya A., Near-infrared estimation of O2 supply and consumption in forearm muscles working at varying intensity, *J. Appl. Physiol.*, Vol. 80, pp. 1279-1284, 1996.

Jöbsis F. F., Noninvasive, infrared monitoring of cerebral and myocardial oxygen sufficiency and circulatory parameters, *Science*, Vol. 198, pp. 1264-1267, 1977.

Lai N., Zhou H., Saidel G. M., Wolf M., McCully K., Gladden L. B. and Cabrera M. E., Modeling oxygenation in venous blood and skeletal muscle in response to exercise using near-infrared spectroscopy, *J. Appl. Physiol.*,Vol. 106, pp. 1858-1874, 2009.

Leff D. R., Warren O. J., Enfield L. C., Gibson A., Athanasiou T., Patten D. K., Hebden J., Yang G. Z. and Darzi A., Diffuse optical imaging of the healthy and diseased breast: A systematic review, *Breast Cancer Res. Treat.*, Vol. 108, pp. 9-22, 2008.

Lin Y., Lech G., Nioka S., Intes X. and Chance B., Noninvasive, low-noise, fast imaging of blood volume and deoxygenation changes in muscles using light-emitting diode continuous-wave imager, *Rev. Sci. Instrum.*, Vol. 73, 3065-3074, 2002.

McCully K. K. and Hamaoka T., Near-Infrared Spectroscopy: What Can It Tell Us about Oxygen Saturation in Skeletal Muscle, *Exercise and sport sciences reviews*, Vol. 28, pp. 123-127, 2000.

Neary J. P., Roberts A. D. W., Leavins N., Harrison M. F., Croll J. C. and Sexsmith J. R., Prefrontal cortex oxygenation during incremental exercise in chronic fatigue syndrome, *Clin. Physiol. Funct. Imaging*, Vol. 28, pp. 364-372, 2008.

Nioka S., Kime R., Sunar U., Im J., Izzetoglu M., Zhang J., Alacam B. and Chance B., A novel method to measure regional muscle blood flow continuously using NIRS kinetics information, *Dynamic Medicine*, Vol. 5, pp. 1-13, 2006.

Pellicer A. and Bravo M. del C., Near-infrared spectroscopy: A methodology-focused review, *Semin. Fetal. Neonat. M.*, Vol. 16, pp. 42-49, 2011.

Prieur F., Berthoin S., Marles A., Blondel N. and Mucci P., Heterogeneity of muscle deoxygenation kinetics during two bouts of repeated heavy exercises, *Eur J. Appl. Physiol.*, Vol. 109, pp. 1047-1057, 2010.

Pogue B. W., Jiang S., Dehghani H., Kogel C., Soho S., Srinivasan S., Song X., Tosteson T. D., Poplack S. P. and Paulsen K. D., Characterization of hemoglobin, water, and NIR scattering in breast tissue: analysis of intersubject variability and menstrual cycle changes, *J. Bio. Opt.*, Vol. 9, pp. 541-552, 2004.

Prasad P. N., Introduction to biophotonics, *John Wiley & Sons Inc.*, 2003.

Quaresima V., Ferrari M., Franceschini M. A., Hoimes M. L. and Fantini S., Spatial distribution of vastus lateralis blood flow and oxyhemoglobin saturation measured at the end of isometric quadriceps contraction by multichannel near-infrared spectroscopy, *J. Bio. Opt.*, Vol. 9, pp. 413-420, 2004.

Quaresima V., Homma S., Azuma K., Shimizu S., Chiarotti F., Ferrari M. and Kagaya A., Calf and shin muscle oxygenation patterns and femoral artery blood flow during dynamic plantar flexion exercise in human, *Eur J. Appl. Physiol.*, Vol. 84, pp. 387-394, 2001.

Quaresima V., Franceschini M. –A., Fantini S., Gratton E. and Ferrari M., Difference in leg muscles oxygenation during treadmill exercise by a new near infrared frequency-domain oximeter, *Proc. SPIE*, Vol. 3194, pp. 116-120, 1998.

Sowa M. G., Leonardi L., Payette J. R., Fish J. S. and Mantsch H. H., Near infrared spectroscopic assessment of hemodynamic changes in the early post-burn period, *Burns*, Vol. 27, pp. 241-249, 2001.

Timinkul A., Kato M., Omori T., Deocaris C. C., Ito A., Kizuka T., Sakairi Y., Nishijima T., Asada T. and Soya H., Enhancing effect of cerebral blood volume by mild exercise in healthy young men: A near-infrared spectroscopy study, *Neurosci. Res.*, Vol. 61, pp. 242-248, 2008.

Tromberg B. J., Cerussi A., Shah N., Compton M., Durkin A., Hsiang D., Butler J. and Mehta R., Diffuse optics in breast cancer: detecting tumors in pre-menopausal women and monitoring neoadjuvant chemotherapy, *Breast Cancer Research*, Vol. 7, pp. 279-285, 2005.

Toronov V., Webb A., Choi J. H., Wolf M., Michalos A., Gratton E. and Hueber D., Investigation of human brain hemodynamics by simultaneous near-infrared spectroscopy and functional magnetic resonance imaging, *Med. Phys.*, Vol. 28, pp. 521-527, 2001.

Vo T. Van, Hammer P. E., Hoimes M. L., Nadgir S. and Fantini S., Mathematical model for the hemodynamic response to venous occlusion measured with near-infrared spectroscopy in the human forearm, *IEEE T. Bio-Med. Eng.*, Vol. 54, pp. 573-584, 2007.

Vernieri F., Tibuzzi F., Pasqualetti P., Rosato N., Passarelli F., Rossini P. M. and Silvestrini M., Transcranial doppler and near-infrared spectroscopy can evaluate the hemodynamic effect of carotid artery occlusion, *Stroke*, Vol. 35, pp. 64-70, 2004.

Villringer A., Planck J., Hock C., Schleinkofer L. and Dirnagl U., Near infrared spectroscopy (NIRS): a new tool to study hemodynamic changes during activation of brain function in human adults, *Neurosci. Lett.*, Vol. 154, pp. 101-104, 1993.

Wang C. -Y., Chuang M. -L., Liang S. -J., Tsai J. -C., Chuang C. -C., Hsieh Y. -S., Lu C. -W., Lee P. -L., and Sun C. -W., Diffuse Optical Multipatch Technique for Tissue Oxygenation Monitoring: Clinical Study in Intensive Care Unit, *IEEE T BIO-MED ENG.*, Vol. 59, pp. 87-94, 2011.

Wu Y. -T., Chiou A. and Sun C. -W., Correlation between tissue oxygenation and erythrocytes elasticity, *J. Biophotonics*, Vol. 4, pp. 224–228, 2011.

Wolf M., Wolf U., Toronov V., Michalos A., Paunescu L. A., Choi J. H. and Gratton E., Different time evolution of oxyhemoglobin and deoxyhemoglobin concentration changes in the visual and motor cortices during functional stimulation: A near-infrared spectroscopy study, *NeuroImage*, Vol. 16, pp. 704-712, 2002.

Yu G., Durduran T., Lech G., Zhou C., Chance B., Mohler III E. R. and Yodh A. G., Time-dependent blood flow and oxygenation in human skeletal muscles measured with noninvasive near-infrared diffuse optical spectroscopies, *J. Bio. Opt.*, Vol. 10, pp. 024027 1-12, 2005.

Zhang Z., Wang B., Gong H., Xu G., Nioka S. and Chance B., Comparisons of muscle oxygenation changes between arm and leg muscles during incremental rowing exercise with near-infrared spectroscopy, *J. Bio. Opt.*, Vol.15, pp. 017007 1-8, 2010.

Zhou C., Choe R., Shah N., Durduran T., Yu G., Durkin A., Hsiang D., Mehta R., Butler J., Cerussi A., Tromberg B. J. and Yodh A. G., Diffuse optical monitoring of blood flow and oxygenation in human breast cancer during early stages of neoadjuvant chemotherapy, *J. Biomed. Opt.*, Vol. 12, pp. 051903 1-11, 2007.

4

How Ozone Treatment Affects Erythrocytes

Sami Aydogan[1] and A. Seda Artis[2]
[1]*Physiology Department, Medical Faculty, Erciyes University*
[2]*Physiology Department, Medical Faculty, Istanbul Medeniyet University*
Turkey

1. Introduction

Blood, a non-Newtonian fluid, is a suspension of formed elements in an aqueous solution of organic molecules, proteins, and salts. The rheological properties of blood are generally well-understood under steady-flow conditions. However, the in vivo flow is unsteady, because of the heart pumping the blood, and blood has to travel through a complex network of vessels of varying geometric qualities (e.g., lumen shape, diameter, single vessels, bifurcations, valves). What's more, the apparent viscosity of blood, which depends on the existing shear forces, is determined by hematocrit, plasma viscosity, and the properties of red blood cells (RBCs) (Baskurt & Meiselman, 2003; Cokelet, 1980; Lipowsky, 2005). In addition to the concentration of cellular elements in blood, the disturbance of flow streamlines depends not only on the concentration of blood cells but also on the behavior of these cells under shear forces (i.e. their rheological properties). RBCs comprise about 45% of the volume of normal blood and are responsible for its complex, scale-dependent rheology. Due to their fluid-filled bag-like structure, RBCs undergo large deformation as they traverse the microcirculation (Baskurt & Meiselman, 2003; Lee & Smith, 2008).

Blood rheology is altered in various conditions: Changes at the level of hematocrit notably lead to variations in hemorheological parameters. Also modifications of the membrane skeletal proteins, the ratio of RBC membrane surface area to cell volume, cell morphology, and cytoplasmic viscosity influence deformability of RBCs. What's more, RBC aggregation is mainly determined by plasma protein composition and surface properties of RBCs (Baskurt & Meiselman, 2003; Lipowsky, 2005). So tissue perfusion may be notably affected by impaired blood fluidity and this may cause to functional deteriorations, especially if the changes had resulted in disturbance of the vascular properties.

The high deformability property of RBCs significantly contributes to aiding blood flow both under bulk flow conditions and in the microcirculation. With diminishing vessel diameter, the particulate nature of blood dominates the resistance to flow. It is now well understood that in addition to blood cell concentration, red cell deformability and aggregation and white blood cell deformability and adhesion to the endothelium are the principal intrinsic factors that affect resistance to flow. Blood cell deformability affects the entrance of blood cells into capillaries. RBCs with reduced deformability in pathological disorders (e.g., sickle cell disease) may be sequestered at the capillary entrance (Lipowsky, 2005).

The aggregation of RBCs is a natural phenomenon affected by high molecular weight molecules, the most important of which is fibrinogen. Erythrocyte aggregation as a reversible

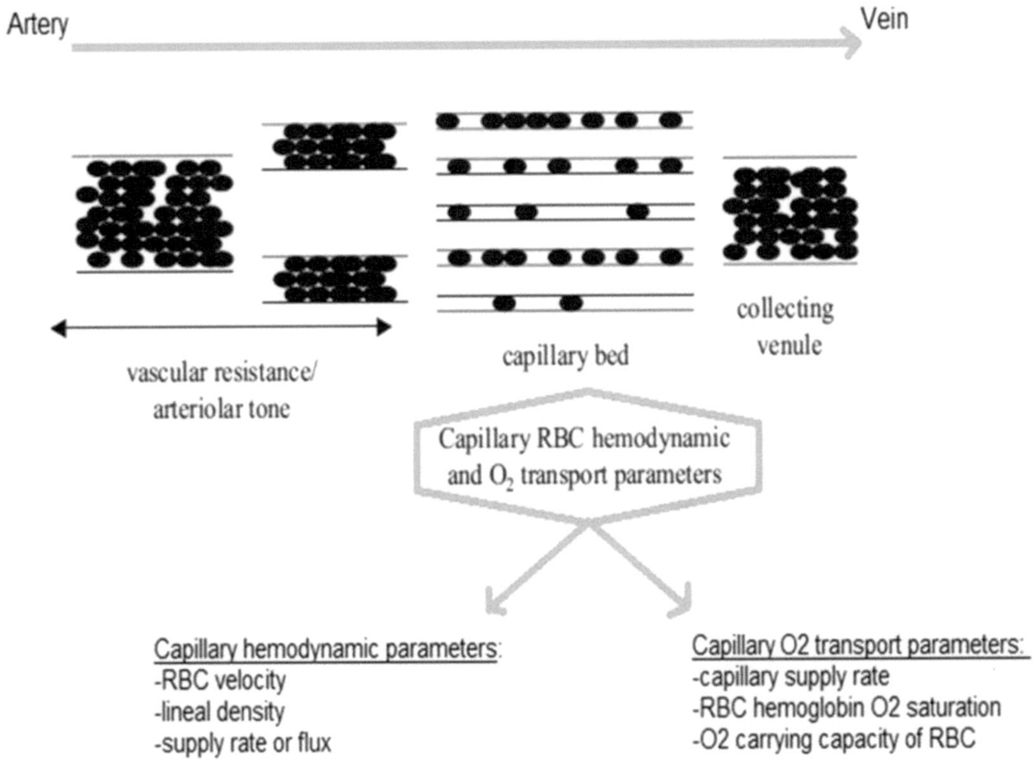

Fig. 1. The above figure, adapted from work of Bateman, clearly shows the interaction and importance of deformability of RBCs for microcirculation. Arteriolar tone establishes the blood flow into an organ, and capillary resistance and rheology factors determine RBC heterogeneity within the capillary bed (Bateman et al., 2003).

dynamic phenomenon can be observed both in vitro and in vivo and is found to be responsible for much of the increase in viscosity at low shear rates. The aggregation combined with yield stress of blood is expected to reduce blood flow compared to that of non-aggregating system (Antonova et al., 2008; Rampling, 1988). The in vivo erythrocyte aggregation observed in certain species at low shear rates is mediated by fibrinogen and other large plasma proteins (Lee & Smith, 2008; Merrill et al., 1966). The term aggregability has been used to express the intrinsic aggregation behavior of RBCs regardless of the properties of the suspending medium (Baskurt & Meiselman, 2003). Although earlier studies suggested that the macromolecular composition of the suspending medium was the only determinant of RBC aggregation, more recent studies have shown that RBC cellular properties also play a very important role in the aggregation process (Armstrong et al., 2001; Baskurt & Meiselman, 2003; Kobuchi et al., 1988; Meiselman, 1993). The process of RBC aggregation can be considered the result of a balance between aggregating and disaggregating forces. Disaggregating forces include fluid shear forces, electrostatic repulsion between cells, and the elastic properties of the cell membrane (Baskurt & Meiselman, 2003; Kobuchi et al., 1988; Mohandas & Chasis, 1993). During red cell aggregation, resistance to flow may decrease with hematocrit reduction or increase due to redistribution of red cells. Blood cell adhesion to the microvessel wall may initiate flow reductions, as, for example, in the case of red cell adhesion to the endothelium in sickle cell disease, or leukocyte adhesion in inflammation (Antonova et al., 2008; Lipowsky, 2005). As strength of aggregation increases, RBCs form rouleaux and then clumps. These clumps frequently became lodged at the capillary entrance and resisted disruption by hydrodynamic forces (Lipowsky, 2005). RBC aggregation is dependent on the magnitude of shearing forces acting on the cells. Increased shear disrupts the aggregates, whereas reduced shear favors aggregation (Baskurt & Meiselman, 2003). RBC aggregation is thus the major determinant of blood viscosity under low shear conditions. Osmotic force arises from the depletion of molecules in the intercellular space where aggregation forces arise naturally as the density of the fluid particles between cells is less than in the surrounding region (Lee & Smith, 2008). So RBC aggregation is accepted as a significant determinant of resistance in venules. However, blood cellular elements other than RBCs have no significant effect on the macroscopic flow properties of blood but may contribute distinctly to blood flow resistance and flow dynamics in the microcirculation (Baskurt & Meiselman, 2003; Kaliviotis et al., 2010; Meiselman & Baskurt, 2006).

The relationship of the RBC's surface area to its volume is evaluated by the osmotic fragility test. The erythrocyte is characterized by a biconcave shape giving it an excess of surface area in relationship to its volume. When a RBC is placed in a hypotonic sodium chloride solution, a net influx of water into the cell will occur. When there is a decrease in the surface area to the cell volume, the osmotic fragility is increased, meaning decreased resistance to hypotonic solutions (and vice versa) (Fernandez-Alberti & Fink, 2000; Mariani et al., 2008).

The rheologic characteristics of blood and its formed elements continue to be of basic science and clinical interest, with numerous publications dealing with topics such as blood and plasma viscosity, RBC aggregation and cell deformability. Alterations of blood's rheologic behavior in pathologic states have been extensively studied, with the findings usually indicating changes assumed to be detrimental to tissue perfusion (e.g., increased RBC aggregation). However, the current literature contains relatively few studies dealing with two important areas: (1) relations between altered rheologic behavior and in vivo hemodynamics; (2) the effects of therapy in those clinical states associated with altered rheologic behavior (Meiselman & Baskurt, 2006).

2. Rheological parameters and pathological conditions

Continuation of the blood flow is essential for the preservation of health and life. Disorders of hemorheology and microcirculatory blood flow play an important role in the pathophysiology and clinical manifestations of a wide range of disease states. There is a large list of causes of microvascular failure (Isbister, 2007). Recent clinical observations have reported that reduced RBC deformability is a common risk factor for circulatory disorders including mainly diabetes, sepsis, malaria, hypertension, sickle cell anemia, ischemic conditions and stroke (Lipowsky, 2007).

In patients with diabetes mellitus there is increased viscosity and enhanced RBC aggregation, which is especially prominent in patients with poor glycemic control (Lacombe et al., 1989; Le Devehat et al., 2001; McKay & Meiselman, 1988). For arterial hypertension the association between blood pressure and blood viscosity should be mentioned. High blood pressure causes elevated hematocrit, plasma viscosity and fibrinogen (Ajmani, 1997; Bogar,

2002; Cicco et al., 1999; Hoieggen et al., 2003; Klein et al., 1995). Severe septic events include misdistribution of blood flow and marked disturbances of microvascular flow leading to tissue hypoperfusion and impaired aggregation and deformability of RBC (Baskurt et al., 1997; Bateman et al., 2003; Condon et al., 2007; Kirschenbaum et al., 2000; Moutzouri et al., 2008; Piagnerelli et al., 2003a; Piagnerelli et al., 2003b; Voerman et al., 1989). Increased aggregation and deformability of RBC is also seen in cerebral and myocardial ischemic conditions as well (Bhavsar & Rosenson, 2010; Bolokadze et al., 2006; Francis, 1991; Huang et al., 1998a; Huang et al., 1998b; Kuke et al., 2001; McHedlishvili et al., 2004).

3. Ozone: Its general effects and use in medicine

Ozone is an inactivated, trivalent (O3) form of oxygen (O2). It is considered one of the most potent oxidants in nature. Ozone was first discovered by chemist Christian Frederick Schonbein in 1840 as a disinfectant (Bocci, 2011).

Ozone was used for the first time to disinfect operating rooms in 1856 and subsequently for water treatment in 1860. It is used to treat battle wounds and other infections during World War I (Bocci, 1996; Bocci, 2006). After the turn of the century, interest began to focus on the uses of ozone in medical therapy. However, it was not until 1932 that ozone was seriously studied by the scientific community, when ozonated water was used as a disinfectant by dentist E.A. Fisch. One of his patients, surgeon Erwin Payr, along with physician P. Aubourg, was the first medical doctor to apply ozone gas through rectal insufflations to treat mucous colitis and fistulae (Bocci, 2006).Major ozonated autohemotherapy was first described in 1954 and consist of ex vivo exposing human blood to a gas mixture composed of therapeutic oxygen and ozone for a short time followed by reinfusion in the donor (Bocci, 2011).

The medical generator of ozone produces it from pure oxygen passing through a high voltage gradient (Bocci, 2006; Li et al., 2007). A gas mixture comprising no less than 95% oxygen and no more than 5% ozone used in medicine is known as medical ozone therapy (Bocci, 2006; Guven et al., 2009). When the gas mixture composed of 95% oxygen and of no more than 5% ozone, is mixed ex vivo, a complex series of physical and chemical processes occur: oxygen dissolved in plasmatic water, almost instantaneously saturates hemoglobin to form oxyhemoglobin and the pO2 increases far higher than physiological level while pCO2 and pH remains fairly constant (Bocci, 1996). But there is not a general consensus regarding the biological effects and possible damage induced by ozone in blood.

It is well known by its toxic effects. Ozone therapy is still a controversial form of alternative therapy. Young children and adults with lung problems are told to stay indoors, because ozone can aggravate allergies, bronchitis, asthma and other health problems. On the other hands, many believe that ozone will help heal them of cancer, heart disease, candida, HIV related problems and a host of other diseases including autoimmune disease, rheumatoid arthritis and low back pain. There are few elements that have been as controversial as ozone, and none that have created such a medical paradox: how can a gas be both dangerous to health as a pollutant, yet can also be used to effectively treat some of humanity's most threatening diseases?

Ozone, when given in lower doses, exerts beneficial effects acting on the oxidant mechanisms (Ajamieh et al., 2002; Chen et al., 2008). In spite of encouraging results obtained with ozone therapy, its clinical use remains controversial due to the scarce knowledge of the mechanisms underlying its therapeutic action and the efficacy in heterogeneous diseases (Ajamieh et al., 2002; Gornicki & Gutsze, 2000). Currently, with reappraisal of ozone therapy, ozone has been utilized worldwide in research and clinical field. It has been used as a therapeutical agent for the treatment of different diseases (Bocci, 2011; Gornicki & Gutsze, 2000; Viebahn-Haensler, 2007).

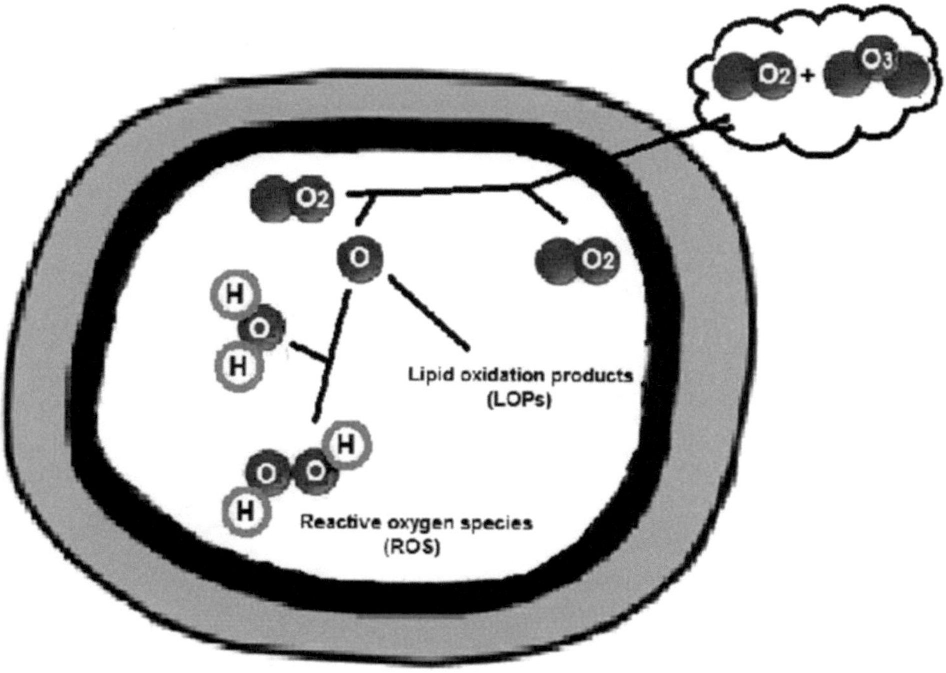

Fig. 2. The fate of oxygen-ozone in the circulation.

Although ozone therapy has drawbacks (as it is intrinsically toxic cannot be breathed, cannot be stored, and must be used with caution and competence), it is used for a wide variety of health problems. There are different methods of ozone therapy in medical practice: direct intra-arterial and intravenous application, rectal insufflations, intramuscular injections, major and minor autohemotherapy, intra-articular injection, ozone bagging, ozonated water, and ozonated oil. Autohemotherapy calls for the removal of venous blood from the patient, and then the ozonated blood is re-introduced into a vein. It is probably the most commonly used type of ozone therapy today. Besides, rectal insufflation method is considered one of the safest (Bocci, 2011; Travagli et al., 2007).

Although ozone has been in use for many years, the dynamic of the events occurring during ozonation of whole human blood have been recently clarified (Bocci & Aldinucci, 2006; Travagli et al., 2006): At a normal gas pressure of 760 mmHg, only 2.0mL of oxygen dissolve in 100mL of water and allows complete oxygenation of hemoglobin. Ozone, one of the strongest oxidants, is 10-fold more soluble than oxygen and, even more important, it reacts immediately with hydrophilic antioxidants present in plasma (Travagli et al., 2007).

Still there is not a general consensus regarding the biological effects and possible damage induced by ozone in blood. The main controversy is due to ozone being an extremely reactive and unstable molecule. However it is well known that the plasma contains a wealth of antioxidants (Travagli et al., 2007). So when erythrocytes are not suspended in saline and their membrane is not deprived of the albumin protection, the antioxidant defense systems of RBCs are activated immediately after the introduction of ozone to the blood.

Ozone also causes a significant reduction in NADH and helps to oxidize cytochrome C. There is a stimulation of production of enzymes which act as free radical scavengers and cell wall protectors: Glulathione peroxidase, catalase, and superoxide dismutase. Production of prostacycline, a vasodilator, is also induced by ozone.

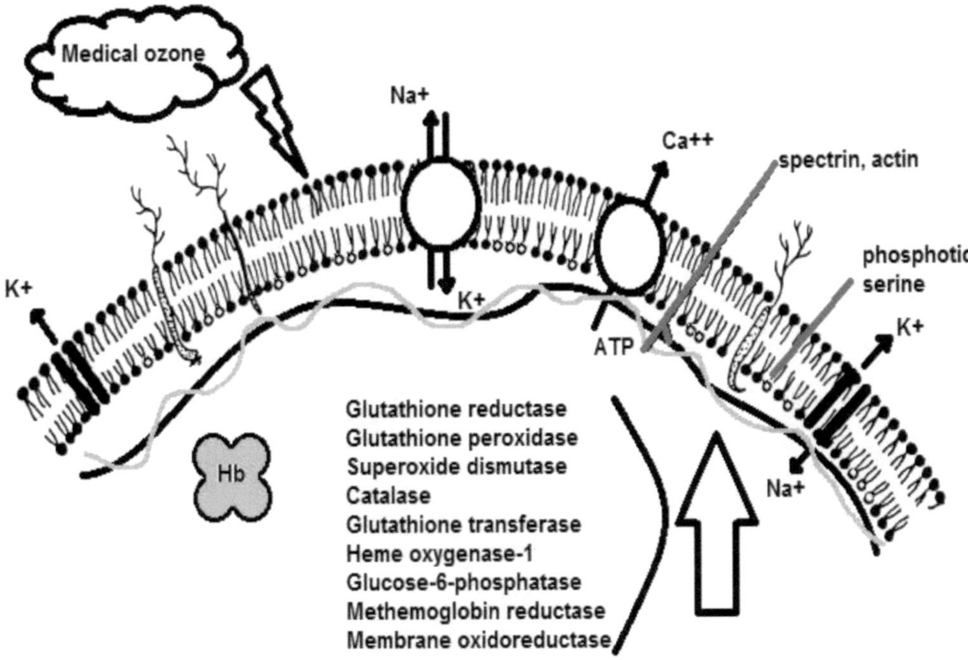

Fig. 3. Ozone possesses the property of stimulating certain antioxidant enzyme systems.

At normal temperature and atmospheric pressure, due to its high solubility and depending upon its relative pressure, some ozone dissolves into the water. But it does not equilibrate with the ozone remaining in the gas phase, unlike oxygen. The reason for this is the immediate interactions between ozone, a potent oxidant, and a variety of molecules present in biological fluids, namely antioxidants, proteins, carbohydrates and, preferentially, polyunsaturated fatty acids (Travagli et al., 2006; Viebahn-Haensler, 2007). Both mono- and polyunsaturated fatty acids and cholesterol, are present in lipoproteins and cellular membranes. Free and bound cysteine, methionine, tyrosine, tryptophane and histine as well as free and protein-bound carbohydrates are among the potential targets (Bocci, 1996).

The reaction of ozone with such a variety of molecular compounds involves: a) an initial stage of reaction in which, some of the ozone dose is unavoidably consumed during oxidation of ascorbic and uric acids, sulphydryl (SH)-groups of proteins and glycoproteins. Although albumin, ascorbic and uric acids tame the harsh reactivity of ozone, they allow this first reaction that is important because it generates reactive oxygen species (ROS), which triggers several biochemical pathways in blood. ROS are neutralized within 0.5-1 minute by the antioxidant system (Bocci, 2011); b) a late stage at which lipid oxidation products (LOPs), such as: peroxyl radical complex mixtures of final products of low molecular weight aldehydes (maloniladdehyde) and alquenales and also, hydrogen peroxide (H2O2). Actually hydrogen peroxide is not a radical oxidant, it is included within ROS. This and the LOPs are responsible for the therapeutic and biological late effects of ozone (Bocci, 1996; Bocci & Aldinucci, 2006). Therefore, the excessive production of oxygen metabolites or inadequate defense to counter their accumulation in the body, with consequent tissue injury, promotes or accelerates the development of multiple pathological processes, being the mechanism of signal transduction for activation or repression of transcription specific genes are the cornerstone of the mechanism of action for modulation of oxidative stress. So only the dose of ozone that is not is consumed by the antioxidants present in plasma stimulates the formation of ROS and LOPs which are responsible for the biological and therapeutic effects of ozone.

It seems obvious that erythrocytes ozonated ex vivo may be modified only for a brief period. Only repeated therapeutic sessions may allow to LOPs to reach the bone-marrow and activate a subtle development at the erythropoietic level, favoring the formation of new RBCs with improved biochemical characteristics, which provisionally were named "supergifted erythrocytes". If this hypothesis is correct, every day, during prolonged ozone therapy, the bone marrow may release a cohort of new RBCs with improved biochemical characteristics (Bocci et al., 2011).

The proposed beneficial effects of ozone therapy does not abruptly stop with the cessation of the therapy but rather persists for 2-3 months, probably in relation to the life-span of the circulating supergifted erythrocytes (Bocci, 2011). During continuing ozone therapy it has been observed that very young RBCs have a significantly higher content of glucose 6-phosphate dehydrogenase (G6PD). This result increase the probability of the postulation that only a cycle of more than 15 treatments could improve an pathology (Bocci et al., 2011).

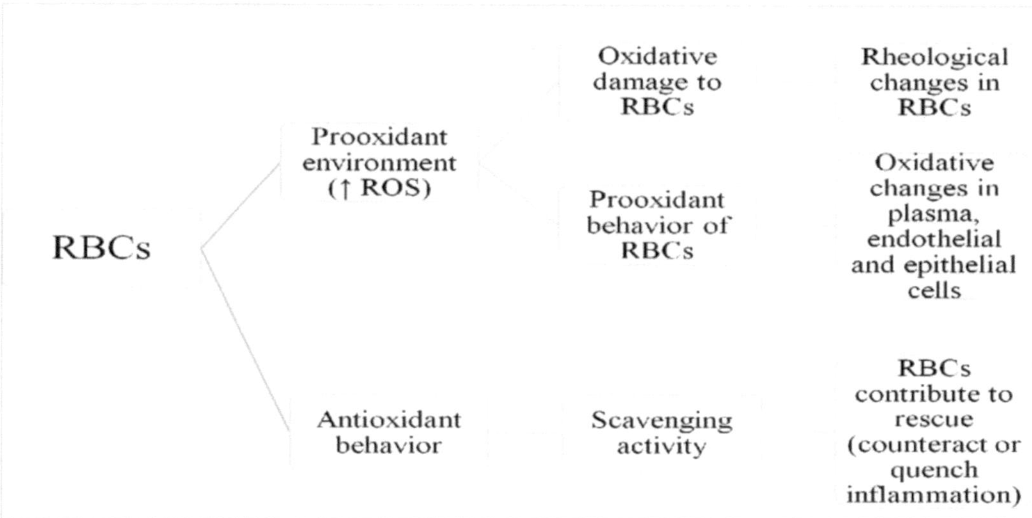

Fig. 4. The oxidant and antioxidant role of RBCs.

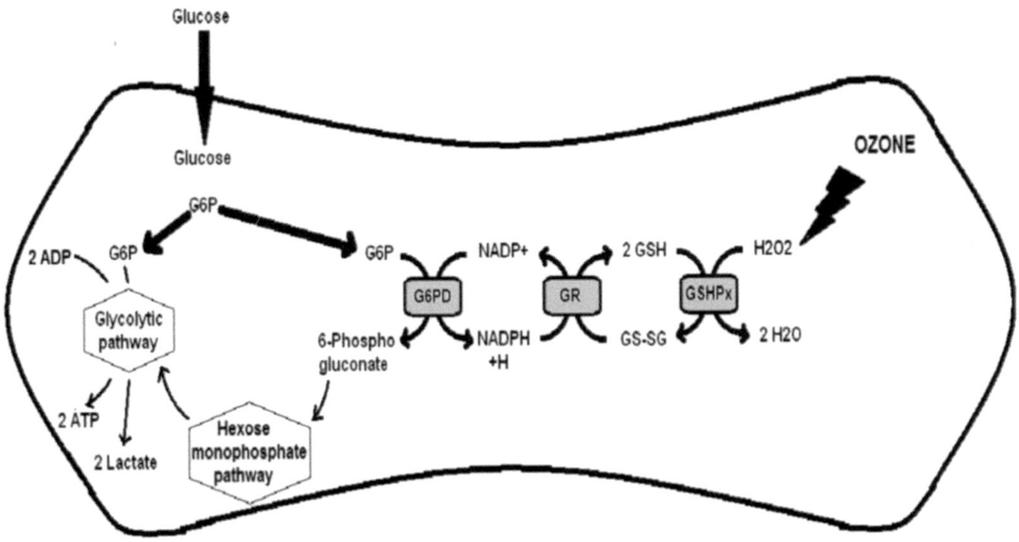

Fig. 5. The action of ozone on the metabolism of red blood cells (G6P: Glucose 6-phosphate; G6PD: Glucose 6-phosphate dehydrogenase; GR: Glutathione reductase; GSHPx: Glutathione peroxidase).

Ozone therapy causes an increase in the RBC glycolysis rate. This leads to the stimulation of 2,3-diphosphoglycerate (2,2-DPG) which leads to an increase in the amount of oxygen released to the tissues. Ozone therapy is avoided in G6PD enzyme deficiency as it acts through this enzyme. Ozone activates the hexose monophosphate pathway by enhancing oxidative carboxylation of pyruvate, stimulating production of ATP (Bateman et al., 2003). Functionally, the oxyhemoglobin sigmoid curve shifts to the right owing to the Bohr effect, i.e. a small pH reduction and a slight increase of 2,3-DPG. The shift to the right is advantageous for improving tissue oxygenation as the chemical bonding of oxygen to hemoglobin is attenuated, facilitating oxygen extraction from ischemic tissues (Bocci et al., 2011).

Above mentioned is the first and immediate reactions following introduction of oxygen-ozone to blood. The second reaction occurs in the bone marrow. When submicromolar amounts of LOPs present in the reinfused blood reach various organs, including the bone marrow, where they can influence the differentiation of the erythroblastic lineage (Bocci, 2011).

Besides, abnormal microvascular oxygen transport indicates that regulatory mechanisms have become dysfunctional and suggests that local cellular environments, as such, have been dramatically altered. The loss of capillary blood flow may potentiate the effects of proinflammatory mediators by increasing their residence time in the microcirculation and tissue (Bateman et al., 2003).

Downstream of the arterioles, microvascular RBC flow is passively distributed throughout the capillary networks and other vascular beds such as the liver sinusoids, according to local vessel resistance (diameter and length) and hemorheologic factors (blood viscosity and RBC deformability). RBCs are forced to deform and travel single file, often separated by plasma gaps, as they pass through vessels that are of smaller diameter then their own. This distinctive microvascular flow behavior maximizes the surface area available for gas exchange between the RBC and the local environment (Bateman et al., 2003).

Flow heterogeneity within capillary beds may have two sources: unequal distribution of RBC supply among arterioles and unique properties of RBC flow in branching networks of capillaries. In determining capillary heterogeneity and functional capillary density, rheologic mechanisms appear to play a greater role than arteriolar heterogeneity, especially at low flow states. These mechanisms are also responsible for the Fahreaus effect, which is the drop in vessel hematocrit along the arteriolar tree to the capillary bed. In the skeletal muscle of septic rats stopped-flow capillaries have lower hematocrit, or lineal density (RBC/mm), than do neighboring flowing capillaries. Neither the implications nor the cause and effect relationship of this phenomenon is clearly understood (Bateman et al., 2003).

4. Hemorheological effects of ozone treatment

In practice, autohemotherapy is the most commonly preferred route for ozone administration; although maybe the safest route to give ozone systemically is rectal insufflations, with almost no side effects. So the effects of ozone on blood cells actually should be investigated with priority. Minor autohaemotherapy involves removing a small amount (usually 10 ml) of the patient's blood from a vein with a hypodermic syringe. The blood is then treated with ozone and oxygen, and given back to the patient with an intramuscular injection. Thus the blood and ozone becomes a type of autovaccine given to the patient that is derived from their own cells, thus forming a unique vaccine that can be very specific and effective in treating the patient's health problem. Major autohemotherapy calls for the removal of 50-100 ml of the patient's blood. Ozone and oxygen are then bubbled into the blood for several minutes, and then the ozonated blood is reintroduced into a vein. Therefore besides giving it for treatment of any pathology involving blood or circulation, during the ozone therapy first blood is prone to the effects of ozone.

The studies investigating the effects of ozone therapy on hematologic/hemodynamic parameters are limited in number and controversial. This is partially because of that many studies on the effects of ozone on blood are conducted under conditions which are not physiologic and looking for the acute effects.

Medical ozone treatment does not practically change neither methemoglobin nor hematocrit levels. Unchanged hematocrit value means no change of the RBC volume due to swelling or lysis. Blood and plasma viscosity decreases due to reduced fibrinogen levels (Bocci, 2002). When high levels of ozone is given there is a minimal loss of K^+, which rapidly returns to normal (Shinriki et al., 1998).

RBC flexibility in mice decreased when ozone given by inhalation (Morgan et al., 1985). Unsurprisingly, loss of deformability reported by the same investigators in a study conducted by ozonating saline-washed RBCs (Morgan et al., 1988). Ozonation of either human whole blood or saline-washed RBCs causes considerable damage. RBCs become quite sensitive to ozone when they are deprived of plasma antioxidants and their membrane has been totally deprived of the albumin protection (Travagli et al., 2007). What's more, in an albumin deprived microenvironment RBCs become echinocytes, that initiates a strong decrease of the deformability (Mrowietz et al., 2008; Wong, 2005). This might be an additional effect to the possible ozone effect on saline-washed RBC. There are three major factors controlling RBC flexibility which should be kept in mind to explain the loss of deformability: Cellular viscosity, the ratio of surface area to volume, and the viscoelastic properties of cell membrane. At high shear rates the internal viscosity of RBC is the major determinant of the deformation; whereas at lower rates of shearing the membrane properties and cell geometry become more important (Baskurt et al., 2009; Bayer & Wasser, 1996).

Following high dose ozone application, Bayer et al. did not find altered deformability of human RBC. They proposed that a direct exposition of RBC (with an intact catalase and/or glutathion system) to ozone leads to an all or nothing effect either leading to no change on RBCs (no influence on elongation) or destroying them (hemolysis) (Bayer & Wasser, 1996). On the other hand, some other researchers have claimed that a slight peroxidation of the RBC membrane induces favorable consequences on cell functions such as increased fluidity of the membrane with enhanced cell deformability (Aydogan et al., 2008; Caglayan & Bayer, 1994; Coppola et al., 2002; Giunta et al., 2001; Rokitansky et al., 1981; Verrazzo et al., 1995). Studies demonstrated that ozone, within the therapeutic range, does not cause oxidation of the RBC membrane (Bocci & Aldinucci, 2006; Cataldo & Gentilini, 2005; Shinriki et al., 1998; Travagli et al., 2006; Travagli et al., 2007). As a consequence, the membrane of RBCs that is shielded by albumin molecules remains intact when we use the therapeutic concentrations of ozone (Travagli et al., 2006; Travagli et al., 2007). The results of our study, where low dose oxygen-ozone mixture rectally applied, showed an increase in RBC deformability proportional to the duration of treatment (Artis et al., 2010).

RBC repels each other because of their negative surface charge from sialic acid residues. At the same time they are attracted by the van der Waals forces, which are electrodynamic in nature. The balance of these two forces determines the most stable arrangement of red cells in an electrolyte solution in the absence of other forces (Fabry, 1987). The cellular properties of RBC determine the cell's intrinsic tendency to aggregate (Baskurt et al., 2009). Ozonation is known to increase the negative charge of the RBC membrane (Travagli et al., 2007). There are studies investigating the effects of ozone application on platelet aggregation, but to our knowledge there is not any study investigating changes in RBC aggregation with ozone treatment in the literature except ours. Following 15 days of treatment with ozone we observed a prominent decrease in RBC aggregation. However, the results were not different than the control group at longer periods of treatment (Artis et al., 2010).

The study of Zimran showed no damaging effects of ozone on red cell enzymes or intermediates. There was only minimal hemolysis that was not different from that caused by routine blood storage (Zimran et al., 2000). This hemolysis may be the result of the reaction of ozone molecules on the red cell membrane lipids, producing secondary ozonides. It is possible that subhemolytic damage to red cells shortens the life span of RBCs reinfusion. However, the number of cells destroyed would be no greater than those destroyed when red cells stored in the blood bank are infused. However as expected washed RBC yield higher values of hemolysis. The degree of hemolysis is lower if the anticoagulant is citrate instead of heparin. This enhanced hemolysis by heparin is probably favored by a concomitant $Ca2+$ influx (Bocci, 2002). On the other hand, exposure of RBC to ozone can result in increased osmotic fragility of the cell membrane (Calabrese et al., 1985; Chan et al., 1977). In accordance with the previous results also we observed a significant increase in osmotic fragility which showed a decrement afterwards with continuing treatment (Artis et al., 2010).

It has recently been discovered that ozone is able to induce an adaptation to oxidative stress or promote an oxidative preconditioning through the increase and preservation of endogenous antioxidant systems (Ajamieh et al., 2002; Bocci, 2011). The adaptation develops after multiple ozone exposures (Ajamieh et al., 2002; Bocci et al., 2007). Prolonged exposure to ozone in aged subjects caused an increase of both ATP and 2,3-DPG in RBCs (Viebahn-Haensler, 2007). Even two weeks of treatment was found enough to induce the adaptation to ozone oxidative stress (Barber et al., 1999; Leon et al., 1998). This adaptation process may explain the changes in RBC aggregation and fragility with extended ozone application; but there was no adaptation in RBC deformability (Artis et al., 2010). It was also observed that 15 days after single dose of ozone application its effect on RBC deformability still persist but lessened (Buckley et al., 1975). Thus when talking about RBC deformability it can be said that there is either a later developing adaptation or it does not exist at all.

An increased negative charge of the membrane accompanied by a lower erythrocyte sedimentation rate together with decreased viscosity may explain an overall improvement of rheologic parameters of ozone therapy (Bocci, 2002).

5. Conclusion

The novelty of ozone therapy is that its functions are directed to restore and improve the metabolism of oxygen, together with sugars and fats to produce energy, through normal metabolic pathways of controlled combustion: Glycolysis, respiratory chain, fatty acid cycle, glucose 6 phosphate dehydrogenase, and oxidative decarboxylation of pyruvate.

Ozone therapy has been used for treatment of a variety of different pathological conditions including peripheral occlusive arterial disease, cerebral ischemia, gangrene, Reynaud's disease, senile dementia, thrombophlebitis, diabetes mellitus, ischemic heart disease, sepsis, etc. Of these, ozone application for superficial infection, burns, dental and intestinal conditions, and circulatory problems seem to have the best potential of cure.

Although ozone treatment is mainly applied as autohemotherapy; and its use is relatively and especially preferred in circulatory disorders (at which both local and systemic routes are preferred) with promising results. However neither its effects nor the mechanisms on blood cells are exactly known. Regarding to ozonation of blood, further research is indicated to delineate the nature of its dynamics and the extent of its effectiveness in (a) the identification of the compounds formed in this process dose and route of application dependently; (b) seeking scientific evidence for metabolic, immunological, endocrine and possibly neurological effects; (c) identification of the possible (and presently known) pathological conditions ozone therapy might be given; and (d) investigating to what extend ozone therapy might be applied in these conditions. With the increasing use of ozone in clinical practice, the RBCs could represent a useful tool to investigate in particular its vascular and hemodynamic effects. More in general, the improvement of clinical laboratory analyses aimed at the evaluation of RBC integrity and function, e.g. morphological/rheological parameters, expression of surface antigens and, RBC redox state, could provide useful information in the clinical practice in the long term.

As a conclusion, ozone treatment seems to have a beneficial effect on RBCs. Nevertheless it should be kept in mind that ozone has different effects after acute or chronic applications on hemorheological properties of RBCs. New controlled studies are needed be conducted on this promising treatment modality. Further studies on this subject are needed.

6. References

Ajamieh, H.; Merino, N.; Candelario-Jalil, E.; Menendez, S.; Martinez-Sanchez, G.; Re, L.; Giuliani, A. & Leon, O.S. (2002). Similar protective effect of ischaemic and ozone oxidative preconditionings in liver ischaemia/reperfusion injury. *Pharmacol Res,* 45,4,pp.333-339.

Ajmani, R.S. (1997). Hypertension and hemorheology. *Clin Hemorheol Microcirc,* 17,6,pp.397-420.

Antonova, N.; Riha, P. & Ivanov, I. (2008). Time dependent variation of human blood conductivity as a method for an estimation of RBC aggregation. *Clin Hemorheol Microcirc,* 39,1-4,pp.69-78.

Armstrong, J.K.; Meiselman, H.J.; Wenby, R.B. & Fisher, T.C. (2001). Modulation of red blood cell aggregation and blood viscosity by the covalent attachment of Pluronic copolymers. *Biorheology,* 38,2-3,pp.239-247.

Artis, A.S.; Aydogan, S. & Sahin, M.G. (2010). The effects of colorectally insufflated oxygen-ozone on red blood cell rheology in rabbits. *Clin Hemorheol Microcirc,* 45,2-4,pp.329-336.

Aydogan, S.; Yapislar, H.; Artis, S. & Aydogan, B. (2008). Impaired erythrocytes deformability in H(2)O(2)-induced oxidative stress: protective effect of L-carnosine. *Clin Hemorheol Microcirc,* 39,1-4,pp.93-98.

Barber, E.; Menendez, S.; Leon, O.S.; Barber, M.O.; Merino, N.; Calunga, J.L.; Cruz, E. & Bocci, V. (1999). Prevention of renal injury after induction of ozone tolerance in rats submitted to warm ischaemia. *Mediators Inflamm,* 8,1,pp.37-41.

Baskurt, O.K.; Boynard, M.; Cokelet, G.C.; Connes, P.; Cooke, B.M.; Forconi, S.; Liao, F.; Hardeman, M.R.; Jung, F.; Meiselman, H.J.; Nash, G.; Nemeth, N.; Neu, B.; Sandhagen, B.; Shin, S.; Thurston, G. & Wautier, J.L. (2009). New guidelines for hemorheological laboratory techniques. *Clin Hemorheol Microcirc,* 42,2,pp.75-97.

Baskurt, O.K. & Meiselman, H.J. (2003). Blood rheology and hemodynamics. *Semin Thromb Hemost,* 29,5,pp.435-450.

Baskurt, O.K.; Temiz, A. & Meiselman, H.J. (1997). Red blood cell aggregation in experimental sepsis. *J Lab Clin Med,* 130,2,pp.183-190.

Bateman, R.M.; Sharpe, M.D. & Ellis, C.G. (2003). Bench-to-bedside review: microvascular dysfunction in sepsis--hemodynamics, oxygen transport, and nitric oxide. *Crit Care,* 7,5,pp.359-373.

Bayer, R. & Wasser, G. (1996). Effects of oxidative stress on erythrocyte deformability. *Proc SPIE* 2678,pp.333–341.

Bhavsar, J. & Rosenson, R.S. (2010). Adenosine transport, erythrocyte deformability and microvascular dysfunction: an unrecognized potential role for dipyridamole therapy. *Clin Hemorheol Microcirc,* 44,3,pp.193-205.

Bocci, V. (1996). Ozone as a bioregulator. Pharmacology and toxicology of ozonotherapy today. . *J Biol Regul Homeost Agents,* 10,2/3,pp.31-53.

Bocci, V., (Ed. (2002). *Oxygen–Ozone Therapy. A critical evaluation*. Kluwer Academic Publisher. Dordrecht.

Bocci, V., (Ed. (2011). *Ozone. A new medical drug*. Springer.

Bocci, V. & Aldinucci, C. (2006). Biochemical modifications induced in human blood by oxygenation-ozonation. *J Biochem Mol Toxicol*, 20,3,pp.133-138.

Bocci, V.; Aldinucci, C.; Mosci, F.; Carraro, F. & Valacchi, G. (2007). Ozonation of human blood induces a remarkable upregulation of heme oxygenase-1 and heat stress protein-70. *Mediators Inflamm*, 2007,pp.26785.

Bocci, V.A. (2006). Scientific and medical aspects of ozone therapy. State of the art. *Arch Med Res*, 37,4,pp.425-435.

Bocci, V.A.; Zanardi, I. & Travagli, V. (2011). Ozone acting on human blood yields a hormetic dose-response relationship. *J Transl Med*, 9,pp.66.

Bogar, L. (2002). Hemorheology and hypertension: not "chicken or egg" but two chickens from similar eggs. *Clin Hemorheol Microcirc*, 26,2,pp.81-83.

Bolokadze, N.; Lobjanidze, I.; Momtselidze, N.; Shakarishvili, R. & McHedlishvili, G. (2006). Comparison of erythrocyte aggregability changes during ischemic and hemorrhagic stroke. *Clin Hemorheol Microcirc*, 35,1-2,pp.265-267.

Buckley, R.D.; Hackney, J.D.; Clark, K. & Posin, C. (1975). Ozone and human blood. *Arch Environ Health*, 30,1,pp.40-43.

Caglayan, S. & Bayer, R. (1994). Effects of oxidative stress on erythrocyte deformability and fragility. *Proc SPIE*, 2082 pp.190-197.

Calabrese, E.J.; Moore, G.S. & Grinberg-Funes, R. (1985). Ozone induced hematological changes in mouse strains with differential levels of erythrocyte G-6-PD activity and vitamin E status. *J Environ Pathol Toxicol Oncol*, 6,2,pp.283-291.

Cataldo, F. & Gentilini, L. (2005). Chemical kinetics measurements on the reaction between blood and ozone. *Int J Biol Macromol*, 36,1-2,pp.61-65.

Chan, P.C.; Kindya, R.J. & Kesner, L. (1977). Studies on the mechanism of ozone inactivation of erythrocyte membrane (Na+ + K+)-activated ATPase. *J Biol Chem*, 252,23,pp.8537-8541.

Chen, H.; Xing, B.; Liu, X.; Zhan, B.; Zhou, J.; Zhu, H. & Chen, Z. (2008). Ozone oxidative preconditioning protects the rat kidney from reperfusion injury: the role of nitric oxide. *J Surg Res*, 149,2,pp.287-295.

Cicco, G.; Vicenti, P.; Stingi, G.D.; Tarallo & Pirrelli, A. (1999). Hemorheology in complicated hypertension. *Clin Hemorheol Microcirc*, 21,3-4,pp.315-319.

Cokelet, G.R. (1980). Rheology and hemodynamics. *Annu Rev Physiol*, 42,pp.311-324.

Condon, M.R.; Feketova, E.; Machiedo, G.W.; Deitch, E.A. & Spolarics, Z. (2007). Augmented erythrocyte band-3 phosphorylation in septic mice. *Biochim Biophys Acta*, 1772,5,pp.580-586.

Coppola, L.; Lettieri, B.; Cozzolino, D.; Luongo, C.; Sammartino, A.; Guastafierro, S.; Coppola, A.; Mastrolorenzo, L. & Gombos, G. (2002). Ozonized autohaemotransfusion and fibrinolytic balance in peripheral arterial occlusive disease. *Blood Coagul Fibrinolysis*, 13,8,pp.671-681.

Fabry, T.L. (1987). Mechanism of erythrocyte aggregation and sedimentation. *Blood*, 70,5,pp.1572-1576.

Fernandez-Alberti, A. & Fink, N.E. (2000). Red blood cell osmotic fragility confidence intervals: a definition by application of a mathematical model. *Clin Chem Lab Med,* 38,5,pp.433-436.

Francis, R.B. (1991). Large-vessel occlusion in sickle cell disease: pathogenesis, clinical consequences, and therapeutic implications. *Med Hypotheses,* 35,2,pp.88-95.

Giunta, R.; Coppola, A.; Luongo, C.; Sammartino, A.; Guastafierro, S.; Grassia, A.; Giunta, L.; Mascolo, L.; Tirelli, A. & Coppola, L. (2001). Ozonized autohemotransfusion improves hemorheological parameters and oxygen delivery to tissues in patients with peripheral occlusive arterial disease. *Ann Hematol,* 80,12,pp.745-748.

Gornicki, A. & Gutsze, A. (2000). In vitro effects of ozone on human erythrocyte membranes: an EPR study. *Acta Biochim Pol,* 47,4,pp.963-971.

Guven, A.; Gundogdu, G.; Vurucu, S.; Uysal, B.; Oztas, E.; Ozturk, H. & Korkmaz, A. (2009). Medical ozone therapy reduces oxidative stress and intestinal damage in an experimental model of necrotizing enterocolitis in neonatal rats. *J Pediatr Surg,* 44,9,pp.1730-1735.

Hoieggen, A.; Fossum, E.; Reims, H. & Kjeldsen, S.E. (2003). Serum uric acid and hemorheology in borderline hypertensives and in subjects with established hypertension and left ventricular hypertrophy. *Blood Press,* 12,2,pp.104-110.

Huang, Y.; Han, L. & Guo, J. (1998a). [Protective effect of selenium on human erythrocyte rheology]. *Zhonghua Yi Xue Za Zhi,* 78,2,pp.101-104.

Huang, Y.M.; Liu, S.; Liu, Y.X.; Lin, D.J.; Duan, C.G.; Li, H.W.; Xiu, R.J. & Zhang, J. (1998b). [An animal experiment and clinical investigation on the protective effect of selenium on the microcirculation induced by free radical damaged RBCs]. *Sheng Li Xue Bao,* 50,3,pp.315-325.

Isbister, J.P., (Ed. (2007). *Hyperviscosity: Clinical disorders.* IOS Press. Amsterdam.

Kaliviotis, E.; Ivanov, I.; Antonova, N. & Yianneskis, M. (2010). Erythrocyte aggregation at non-steady flow conditions: a comparison of characteristics measured with electrorheology and image analysis. *Clin Hemorheol Microcirc,* 44,1,pp.43-54.

Kirschenbaum, L.A.; Aziz, M.; Astiz, M.E.; Saha, D.C. & Rackow, E.C. (2000). Influence of rheologic changes and platelet-neutrophil interactions on cell filtration in sepsis. *Am J Respir Crit Care Med,* 161,5,pp.1602-1607.

Klein, W.; Eber, B.; Dusleag, J.; Gasser, R.; Fruhwald, F.M.; Schumacher, M.; Zweiker, R. & Stoschitzky, K. (1995). [Hypertension and hemorheology]. *Wien Med Wochenschr,* 145,15-16,pp.355-357.

Kobuchi, Y.; Ito, T. & Ogiwara, A. (1988). A model for rouleaux pattern formation of red blood cells. *J Theor Biol,* 130,2,pp.129-145.

Kuke, D.; Donghua, L.; Xiaoyan, S. & Yanjun, Z. (2001). Alteration of blood hemorheologic properties during cerebral ischemia and reperfusion in rats. *J Biomech,* 34,2,pp.171-175.

Lacombe, C.; Lelievre, J.C.; Bucherer, C. & Grimaldi, A. (1989). Activity of Daflon 500 mg on the hemorheological disorders in diabetes. *Int Angiol,* 8,4 Suppl,pp.45-48.

Le Devehat, C.; Khodabandehlou, T. & Vimeux, M. (2001). Impaired hemorheological properties in diabetic patients with lower limb arterial ischaemia. *Clin Hemorheol Microcirc,* 25,2,pp.43-48.

Lee, J. & Smith, N.P. (2008). Theoretical modeling in hemodynamics of microcirculation. *Microcirculation,* 15,8,pp.699-714.

Leon, O.S.; Menendez, S.; Merino, N.; Castillo, R.; Sam, S.; Perez, L.; Cruz, E. & Bocci, V. (1998). Ozone oxidative preconditioning: a protection against cellular damage by free radicals. *Mediators Inflamm*, 7,4,pp.289-294.

Li, L.J.; Yang, Y.G.; Zhang, Z.L.; Nie, S.F.; Li, Z.; Li, F.; Hua, H.Y.; Hu, Y.J.; Zhang, H.S. & Guo, Y.B. (2007). Protective effects of medical ozone combined with traditional Chinese medicine against chemically-induced hepatic injury in dogs. *World J Gastroenterol*, 13,45,pp.5989-5994.

Lipowsky, H.H. (2005). Microvascular rheology and hemodynamics. *Microcirculation*, 12,1,pp.5-15.

Lipowsky, H.H., (Ed. (2007). *Blood rheology aspects of the microcirculation*. IOS Press. Amsterdam.

Mariani, M.; Barcellini, W.; Vercellati, C.; Marcello, A.P.; Fermo, E.; Pedotti, P.; Boschetti, C. & Zanella, A. (2008). Clinical and hematologic features of 300 patients affected by hereditary spherocytosis grouped according to the type of the membrane protein defect. *Haematologica*, 93,9,pp.1310-1317.

McHedlishvili, G.; Lobjanidze, I.; Momtselidze, N.; Bolokadze, N.; Varazashvili, M. & Shakarishvili, R. (2004). About spread of local cerebral hemorheological disorders to whole body in critical care patients. *Clin Hemorheol Microcirc*, 31,2,pp.129-138.

McKay, C.B. & Meiselman, H.J. (1988). Osmolality-mediated Fahraeus and Fahraeus-Lindqvist effects for human RBC suspensions. *Am J Physiol*, 254,2 Pt 2,pp.H238-249.

Meiselman, H. (1993). Red blood cell role in RBC aggregation: 1963–1993 and beyond. *Clin Hemorheol* 13,pp.575–592.

Meiselman, H.J. & Baskurt, O.K. (2006). Hemorheology and hemodynamics: Dove andare? *Clin Hemorheol Microcirc*, 35,1-2,pp.37-43.

Merrill, E.W.; Gilliland, E.R.; Lee, T.S. & Salzman, E.W. (1966). Blood rheology: effect of fibrinogen deduced by addition. *Circ Res*, 18,4,pp.437-446.

Mohandas, N. & Chasis, J.A. (1993). Red blood cell deformability, membrane material properties and shape: regulation by transmembrane, skeletal and cytosolic proteins and lipids. *Semin Hematol*, 30,3,pp.171-192.

Morgan, D.L.; Dorsey, A.F. & Menzel, D.B. (1985). Erythrocytes from ozone-exposed mice exhibit decreased deformability. *Fundam Appl Toxicol*, 5,1,pp.137-143.

Morgan, D.L.; Furlow, T.L. & Menzel, D.B. (1988). Ozone-initiated changes in erythrocyte membrane and loss of deformability. *Environ Res*, 45,1,pp.108-117.

Moutzouri, A.G.; Athanassiou, G.A.; Dimitropoulou, D.; Skoutelis, A.T. & Gogos, C.A. (2008). Severe sepsis and diabetes mellitus have additive effects on red blood cell deformability. *J Infect*, 57,2,pp.147-151.

Mrowietz, C.; Hiebl, B.; Franke, R.P.; Park, J.W. & Jung, F. (2008). Reversibility of echinocyte formation after contact of erythrocytes with various radiographic contrast media. *Clin Hemorheol Microcirc*, 39,1-4,pp.281-286.

Piagnerelli, M.; Boudjeltia, K.Z.; Brohee, D.; Piro, P.; Carlier, E.; Vincent, J.L.; Lejeune, P. & Vanhaeverbeek, M. (2003a). Alterations of red blood cell shape and sialic acid membrane content in septic patients. *Crit Care Med*, 31,8,pp.2156-2162.

Piagnerelli, M.; Boudjeltia, K.Z.; Vanhaeverbeek, M. & Vincent, J.L. (2003b). Red blood cell rheology in sepsis. *Intensive Care Med*, 29,7,pp.1052-1061.

Rampling, M.W., (Ed. (1988). *Red cell aggregation and yield stress* CRC Press, Boca Raton, FL.

Rokitansky, O.; Rokitansky, A.; Steiner, I.; Trubel, W.; Viebahn, R. & Washuttl, J. (1981). *Proceedings of 5th OzoneWorld Congress*, Germany, Wasser Berlin GmbH.

Shinriki, N.; Suzuki, T.; Takama, K.; Fukunaga, K.; Ohgiya, S.; Kubota, K. & Miura, T. (1998). Susceptibilities of plasma antioxidants and erythrocyte constituents to low levels of ozone. *Haematologia (Budap)*, 29,3,pp.229-239.

Travagli, V.; Zanardi, I. & Bocci, V. (2006). A realistic evaluation of the action of ozone on whole human blood. *Int J Biol Macromol*, 39,4-5,pp.317-320.

Travagli, V.; Zanardi, I.; Silvietti, A. & Bocci, V. (2007). A physicochemical investigation on the effects of ozone on blood. *Int J Biol Macromol*, 41,5,pp.504-511.

Verrazzo, G.; Coppola, L.; Luongo, C.; Sammartino, A.; Giunta, R.; Grassia, A.; Ragone, R. & Tirelli, A. (1995). Hyperbaric oxygen, oxygen-ozone therapy, and rheologic parameters of blood in patients with peripheral occlusive arterial disease. *Undersea Hyperb Med*, 22,1,pp.17-22.

Viebahn-Haensler, R., (Ed. (2007). *The Use of Ozone in Medicine*. ODREI Publishers. Iffezheim, Germany.

Voerman, H.J.; Fonk, T. & Thijs, L.G. (1989). Changes in hemorheology in patients with sepsis or septic shock. *Circ Shock*, 29,3,pp.219-227.

Wong, P. (2005). A hypothesis of the disc-sphere transformation of the erythrocytes between glass surfaces and of related observations. *J Theor Biol*, 233,1,pp.127-135.

Zimran, A.; Wasser, G.; Forman, L.; Gelbart, T. & Beutler, E. (2000). Effect of ozone on red blood cell enzymes and intermediates. *Acta Haematol*, 102,3,pp.148-151.

5

Regulation of Renal Hemodyamics by Purinergic Receptors in Angiotensin II – Induced Hypertension

Martha Franco[1], Rocío Bautista-Pérez[1] and Oscar Pérez-Méndez[2]
[1]*Nephrology Department, Instituto Nacional de Cardiologia "Ignacio Chavez",*
[2]*Molecular Biology Department, Instituto Nacional de Cardiologia "Ignacio Chavez",*
México

1. Introduction

1.1 Effect of purinergic receptors activation on the regulation of renal hemodynamics

Extracellular ATP participates in several physiological processes such as neurotransmission, modulation of vascular tone, contraction of smooth muscle cells, aggregation of platelets and signal transmission (Burnstock, 2006). ATP, and its metabolite adenosine are characterized by their vasoactive properties in several arterial beds, including the renal microcirculation. Purinergic receptors (P1 and P2) are expressed in the cortex and medulla of kidney; P1 are mainly activated by adenosine (ADO) and P2 receptors are activated by ATP. Both, P1 and P2 receptors participate in the in the regulation of vascular tone and hemodynamics in the kidney microvasculature, and have an important role in the tubuloglomerular feedback mechanism. (Schnermann & Levine, 2003; Navar, 1998; Mitchell & Navar, 1993; Inscho, 2001).

Purinergic receptors P1 include four receptors subtypes, A1, A2a, A2b, and A3 (Inscho et al., 1992); A1 and A3 receptors are coupled to Gi proteins, inhibiting adenyl cyclase when these receptors are activated by its agonists, with the consequent decrease of intracellular cAMP. High affinity A1 receptors are constitutively activated in the renal vessels and induce vasoconstriction whereas the location and functional role of the A3 receptors in the kidney remains unclear. In contrast, the A2a and A2b receptors are coupled to Gs protein and interaction with exogenous adenosine produces systemic vasodilation in most of vascular beds, but paradoxical vasoconstriction in the kidney microcirculation.

In addition, adenosine has been implicated in the regulation of glomerular filtration rate and activation of the tubuloglomerular feedback mechanism (Franco, et al., 1989; Schnermann & Levine, 2003). In this regard, exogenous adenosine induces an increase in afferent and efferent resistances, which results in a fall of glomerular blood flow, glomerular capillary pressure, and ultrafiltration coefficient, leading to a decrease in single nephron glomerular filtration rate (Franco et al., 1996; Osswald, 1984). Concerning the tubuloglomerular feedback (TGF) mechanism, administration of A1 receptors blockers prevented the glomerular capillary pressure decrease (or single nephron glomerular filtration rate) induced by the perfusion to the macula densa; these results indicate an inhibition of the TGF mechanism. In contrast, adenosine and its analogues markedly increased the glomerular capillary pressure after perfusion of the macula densa, thus enhancing the response of the TGF mechanism, an effect that seems to be related to the activation of adenosine A1 receptors. In this regard, adenosine is required for elicit a normal TGF response (Schnermann & Levine, 2003).

ATP Purinergic receptors include two types of membrane proteins, P2X and P2Y. These receptors have important structural differences; seven subtypes have been described, P2X 1-7, and these receptors are non-selective cation channels composed by two transmembrane domains that facilitate the entry of extracellular calcium. P2Y receptors include eight subtypes, P2Y 1, 2, 4, 6, 11, 12, 13, and 14; these receptors are G protein-coupled proteins with transmembrane domains associated to phospholipase C that induces the elevation of cytosolic calcium from the intracellular stores (Burnstock, 2007; Guang et al., 2007). The effect of P2 receptors depends of the cell type; P2X receptors are mainly located in the smooth muscle cells and P2Y receptor are predominate in the endothelial cells. P2X receptor activation in the smooth muscle cells produces renal vasoconstriction; in the endothelial cells only P2X4 has been described as able to induce vasodilation. P2Y receptor activation in the endothelial cells induces vasodilation, and by release of nitric oxide or prostaglandin I_2 (Wihlborg et al., 2003), whereas in the smooth muscle cells induces vasoconstriction through increasing intracellular calcium release.

The ATP vascular effects are difficult to evaluate due to the degradation of this molecule to adenosine by ectonucleotidases, as well as to the enhanced endothelial production of nitric oxide induced by ATP. The nucleotide induces renal vasoconstriction in rabbits and rats; infusion of ATP produces an inconsistent decrease in the glomerular capillary pressure that becomes a sustained vasoconstriction under blockade of adenosine receptors (Mitchell & Navar, 1993). However in dogs, infusion of ATP into the renal artery produces an increase in renal blood flow; in this model, when nitric oxide production is blockaded before the ATP infusion, the renal vasodilation is impaired. These changes are due to the differential effect of P2Y receptors stimulation on endothelial and smooth muscle cells; P2Y receptors enhance the production of nitric oxide by endothelial cells, but the direct activation of P2X receptors in the vascular smooth muscle cells induce vasoconstriction in the renal microcirculation (Inscho, 2009). On the other hand, ATP inhibits the tubuloglomerular feedback response; the mechanism of such inhibition is still unclear but it has been demonstrated that it is not mediated by degradation of the nucleotide to adenosine (Mitchell & Navar, 1993). In other words, it likely that extracellular ATP contributes to the regulation of TGF responsiveness.

In the isolated juxtamedullary nephron preparation, ATP induces an initial vasoconstriction of the afferent arterioles (Inscho et al., 1995; Inscho et al.,1996) that wanes and finally remains a residual vasoconstriction, as observed in "in vivo" studies; the blockade of adenosine receptors increases the ATP-mediated vasoconstriction. The ATP vasoconstrictor effect was maintained during the blockade of nitric oxide, supporting the notion that stimulation of P2Yreceptors induce an initial vasoconstriction that is counterbalanced by a later NO release, resulting in a transient vasoconstriction induced by ATP (Inscho et al., 1994). In contrast to the effects on afferent arterioles, the efferent arteriole does not respond to ATP, which suggests a low number of P2 receptors (Inscho et al., 1994; Chan et al, 1998).

2. Renal hemodynamics in the Ang II-infused hypertensive rat

Angiotensin II-induced hypertension is characterized by elevated intrarenal Ang II levels, renal vasoconstriction and renal injury (Zou et al., 1996; Shao et al., 2009; Franco et al., 2001, Johnson et al., 1992, Arendshorst et al., 1999). As previously observed in this model, systolic blood pressure increased through the 14 days infusion period and was associated with a marked proteinuria (Figure 1), as well as a dramatic fall in urinary nitrate excretion.

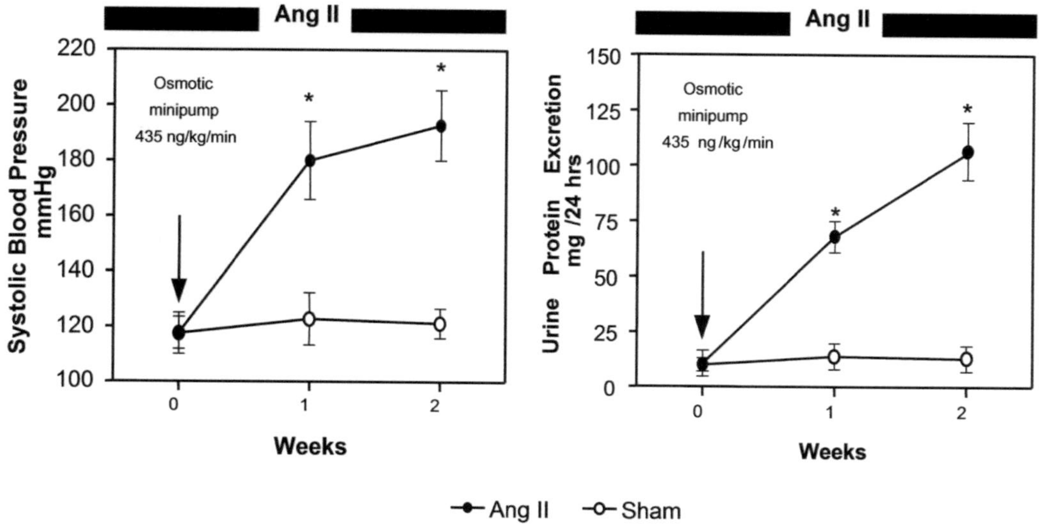

Fig. 1. Follow up of systolic blood pressure and proteinuria during 14 days after Ang II was infused by an osmotic minipump (modified from Franco et al. 2001).

This hemodynamic pattern in the Ang II-induced hypertension is similar to the changes produced by acute infusion of the peptide (Blantz et al., 1976). After 14 days of Ang II infusion, glomerular hemodynamics is characterized by intense renal vasoconstriction, with a decrease in total glomerular filtration rate. At the single nephron level, a marked elevation of afferent resistance and a mild increase of efferent resistance are observed; the increase in resistances lead to a fall in glomerular plasma flow and ultrafiltration coefficient (Kf); as a result, the single nephron glomerular filtration rate was markedly reduced as a consequence of the concomitant decrease in Kf as seen in Figure 2.

A fall in the production of renal vasodilators such as nitric oxide is suggested by the marked decrease in urinary nitrites/nitrates during the Ang II infusion, which also contributes to the renal vasoconstriction. Consistent with the reduction of urinary nitrites, it has been reported that the infusion of Ang II results in an attenuated immunostaining of nitric oxide synthase 1 (NOS1) in the macula densa and of NOS 3 in the outer and inner medulla (Lombardi et al., 1999).

In addition, a marked structural injury is associated to the Ang II-induced hypertension that may be responsible for the alteration of renal hemodynamics; proliferation of smooth muscle cells with an increased thickness of the afferent arteriole is observed. Even if these alterations are common findings in hypertension, Ang II also induces smooth muscle proliferation by itself. However, the most important renal alterations induced by Ang II are the increase of smooth muscle α-actin expression by mesangial cells in spite of minimal glomerular cell proliferation, a tubulointerstitial damage characterized by myofibroblasts adjacent to the peritubular capillary network, fibrosis by focal deposition of collagen type IV, as well as an infiltration of monocytes and interstitial deposit of osteopontin (Johnson et al., 1992). A minimal focal tubular cells injury and proliferation, was also observed (Johnson et al., 1992; Ozawa et al., 2007).

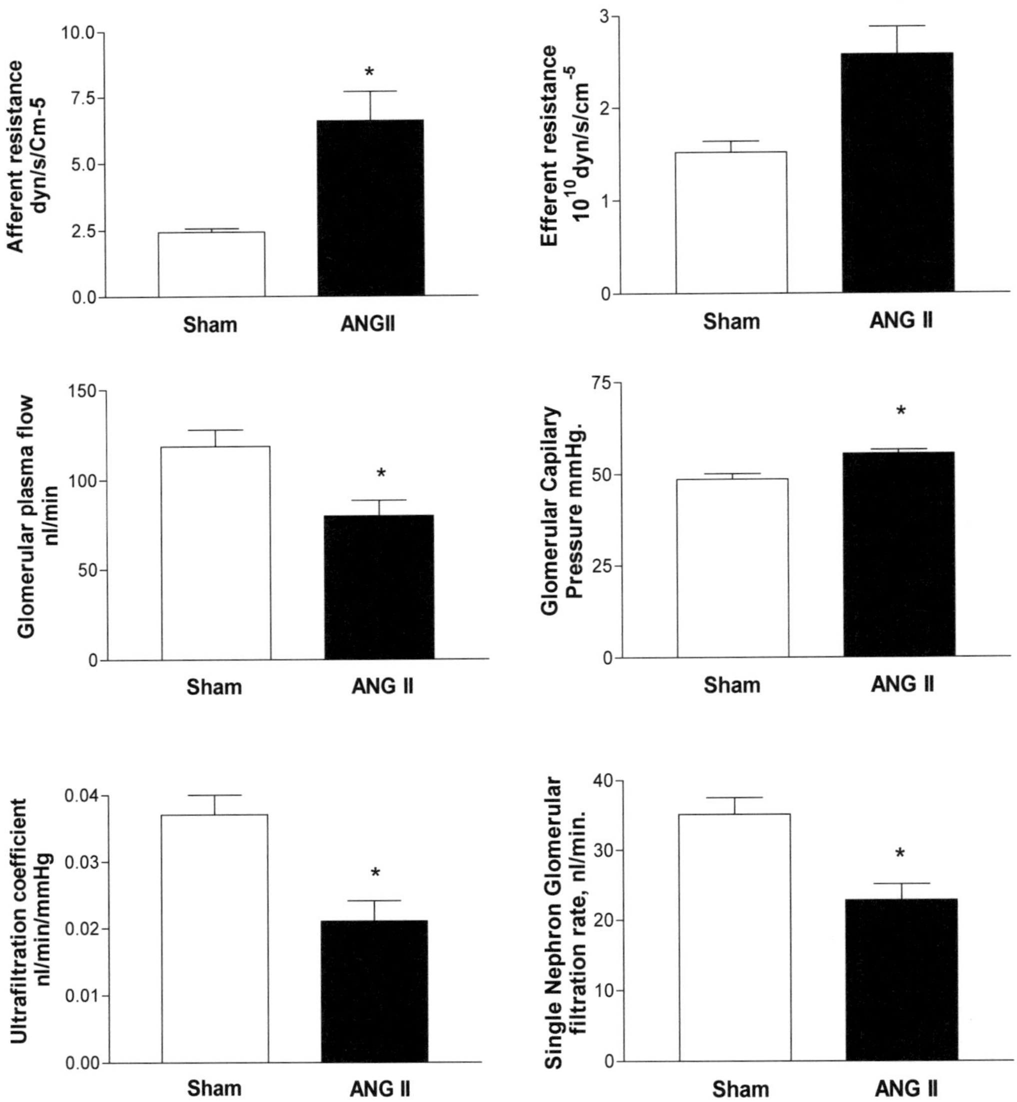

Fig. 2. Glomerular hemodynamics in Sham and Ang II hypertensive rats. The effects of angiotensin are shown in afferent and efferent resistances, glomerular plasma flow, glomerular capillary pressure, ultrafiltration coefficient and single nephron glomerular filtration rate (modified from Franco et al. 2001).

In this regard, relevant importance has been attributed to the production of cytokines, growth factors and angiotensin II produced by the interstitial inflammatory cells, that enhances intrarenal Ang II and induces renal cortical vasoconstriction (Rodriguez-Iturbe et al., 2001; Suzuky et al., 2003; Ruiz-Ortega et al., 2003; Franco el at., 2006). In addition to the direct effects of Ang II on the renal microcirculation, several vasoactive compounds appears to contribute to elevate the renal vascular resistance, including endothelin, 20-HETE and asymmetric dimethyl arginine, as well as ATP and adenosine (Sasser et al., 2002; Lai et al., 2009).

3. Participation of adenosine receptors in the renal vasoconstriction of Ang II-infused hypertensive rat

Several conditions that induce the elevation of Ang II concentrations also enhance the vasoconstrictor response of the kidney to adenosine (Hall & Granger, 1986; Hansen et al., 2003; Weihprecht et al., 1994; Nishiyama et al., 2001). Furthermore, various studies suggest that Ang II-induced ischemia results in the novo formation of adenosine. In this context, an important factor to take in consideration is that adenosine is a vasoactive metabolite of ATP, and the elevation of blood pressure by Ang II results in a high interstitial renal concentrations of ATP.

The synergic interaction between Ang II and adenosine to induce renal vasoconstriction is well recognized (Hall et al., 1985; Weihprecht et al., 1994) and it is essential in the regulation of renal hemodynamics and tubuloglomerular feedback (Osswald et al., 1977). Nevertheless, the mechanisms involved in such synergic interaction have not been completely elucidated; several studies suggest that under acute changes in the concentration of the corresponding agonists, the degree of activation of Ang II AT1 or adenosine A1 receptors determines the magnitude of the constrictor response of the renal vasculature (Weihprecht et al., 1994). Furthermore, the synergism seems partially mediated by A1 receptors, since in the adenosine A1 knockout mice AT1 and A2a receptors remained unchanged, but the vascular response to Ang II in the kidney was diminished (Hansen et al., 2003). Taking into account that the local renal adenosine concentrations could be the factor that contributes to the interaction with Ang II (Franco et al., 2008), we measured de interstitial adenosine concentrations in the cortex of sham-control and Ang II-treated rats. Ang II doses were 435, 260 or 130 ng/kg/min, and as observed in Figure 3, only the higher dose significantly increased both tissue content and interstitial concentrations. It has been proposed that the renal vasoconstriction and reduced glomerular filtration rate observed in the Ang II model results from a fall in glomerular plasma flow and Kf (Franco et al., 2008), as a consequence of the Ang II administration. Indeed, our results obtained in the micropuncture experiments clearly demonstrate the vasoconstriction after 14 days of infusion with Ang II. In this regard, Zou et al. (Zou et al., 1996) demonstrated that after 14 days of treatment, Ang II was elevated in the kidney; the renal concentration of Ang II may be attributed to the accumulation of the exogenous peptide, but endogenous angiotensin was also elevated. Since adenosine content and interstitial concentration of adenosine are elevated, the interaction between both vasoactive compounds is certain. In addition, when we infused the specific A1 adenosine receptor blocker DPCPX, the blood pressure remained unchanged, and the renal hemodynamic alterations induced by Ang II were completely reversed. Under these conditions, only the glomerular capillary pressure remained elevated, suggesting an impairment of autoregulation, which allowed the transmission of the systemic pressure to the glomeruli (Figure 4). These experiments demonstrate the contribution of adenosine receptor in the renal vasoconstriction by temporal infusion of Ang II.

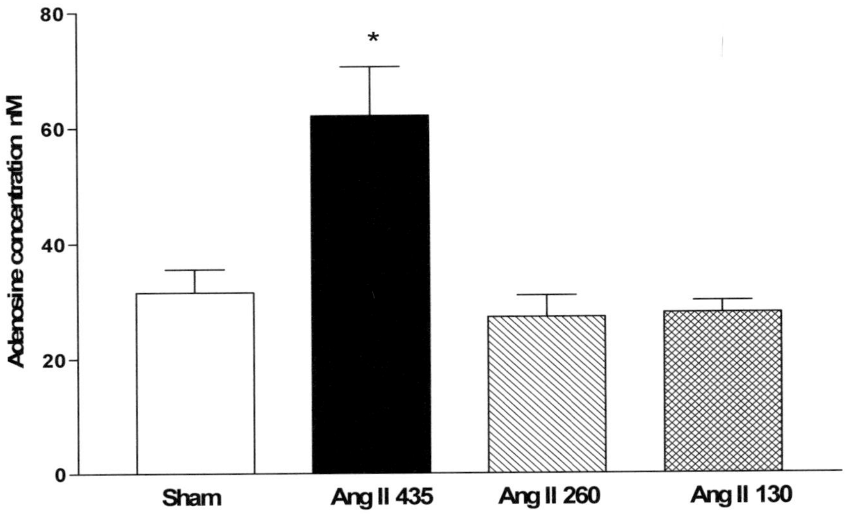

Fig. 3. Interstitial adenosine concentration in the renal cortex of Sham and Ang II-treated rats Ang II doses were 435, 260 or 130 ng•kg^{-1}•min^{-1} * p<0,001 vs. Sham, and vs. Ang II 260 and 130 ng•kg^{-1}•min^{-1}, (modified from Franco et al. 2008).

To evaluate the mechanism involved in the increased concentration of adenosine in the kidney of Ang II hypertensive rats, we evaluated the enzymes involved in the metabolism of adenosine. On one hand, the 5´nucleotidase catalyzes the conversion of adenine nucleotides to adenosine in the extracellular compartment from renal sympathetic nerve terminals, renal endothelial cells, renal vascular smooth muscle cells and/or epithelial cells (Gordon et al., 1989; Jackson et al., 2007). On the other hand, adenosine deaminase is responsible of the degradation of ADO to inosine, which has not vasoactive properties. When the activities of 5´-nucleotidase and adenosine deaminase were investigated, the enzyme located at cytosol as well as that on the membrane were separated to evaluate the participation of both fractions. Despite the lack of changes of 5´-nucleotidase activity, adenosine deaminase activity was significantly higher in the membrane fraction from the Sham-control group that in those from the Ang II-treated rats, without changes in the cytosol fraction (Figure 5).

Despite a lack of changes in the cytosolic and membrane activity of the 5´-nucleotidase between control and Ang II groups, the adenosine deaminase activity was decreased in the Ang II group; these changes were associated to a decrease in protein and mRNA levels of adenosine deaminase.

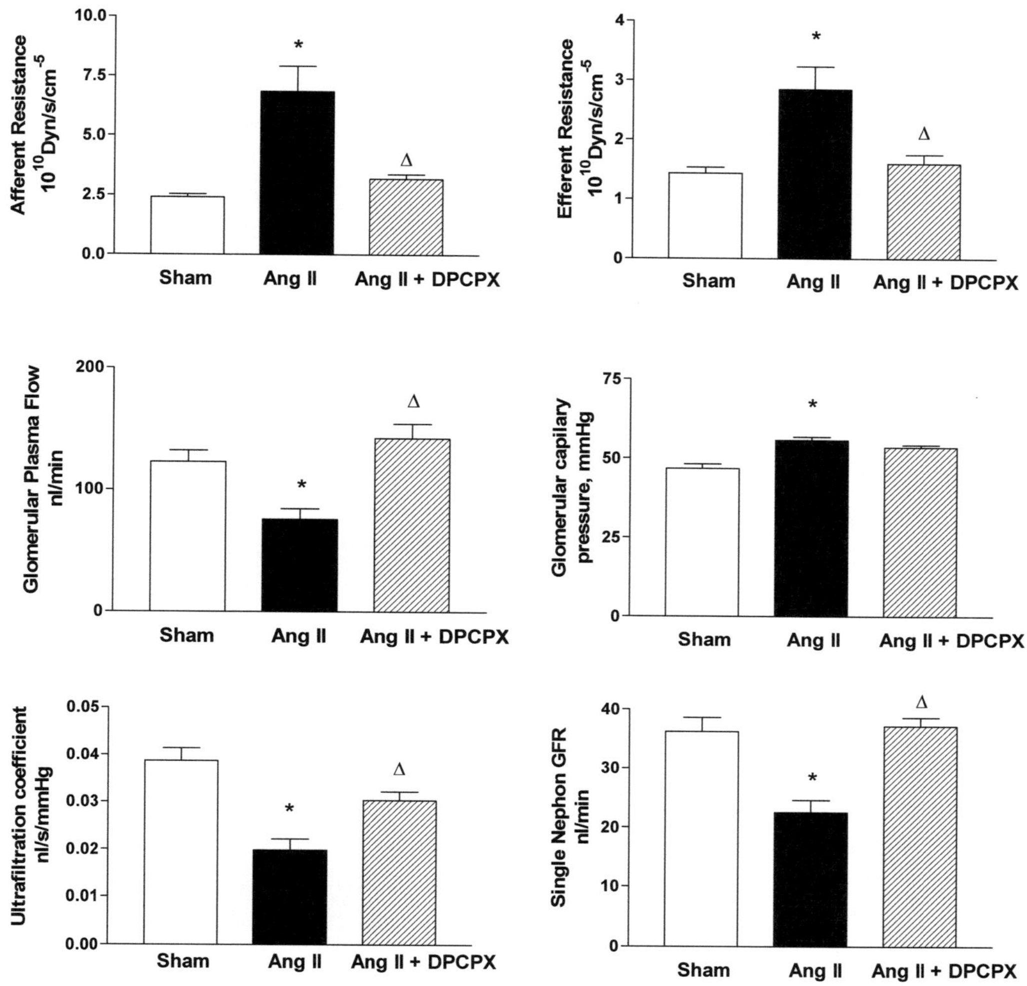

Fig. 4. Afferent and efferent resistances, glomerular plasma flow, glomerular capillary pressure, ultrafiltration coefficient and single nephron GFR in Sham, Ang II hypertensive rats and Ang II with infusion of the adenosine A1 blocker DPCPX. *p< 0.01 vs. Sham; △ p< 0.01 vs. Ang II, (modified from Franco et al. 2008).

These data are in agreement with the adenosine concentration found in the tissue and with microdialysis determinations in Ang II treated animals (Franco et al., 2008). In addition, since ecto-and intracellular enzymes were separated in this study, the changes in the ecto-adenosine deaminase suggest that the increase of interstitial adenosine concentrations could be attained through both, the decreased activity of ecto-adenosine deaminase, and an increased production of adenosine. In this regard, studies by Dietrich et al.,((Dietrich et al., 1991) have demonstrated that adenosine can be synthetized in the extracellular compartment through the breakdown of ATP. The ATP is released from circulating erythrocytes when luminal partial pressure of O_2 falls in the arterioles, as happens in the Ang II-mediated hypertensive model (Welch et al., 2005). Moreover, microvascular endothelial cells and basolateral membranes from the proximal tubule have high activity of extracellular ecto-nucleotidase, which degrades adenine nucleotides to adenosine (Jackson et al., 2001; Jackson et al., 2007). The adenosine increase in renal tissue observed in the Ang II-induced hypertension is probably the result of a significant increase of local nucleotidase, and a reduction of ecto-adenosine deaminase (Franco et al., 2008).

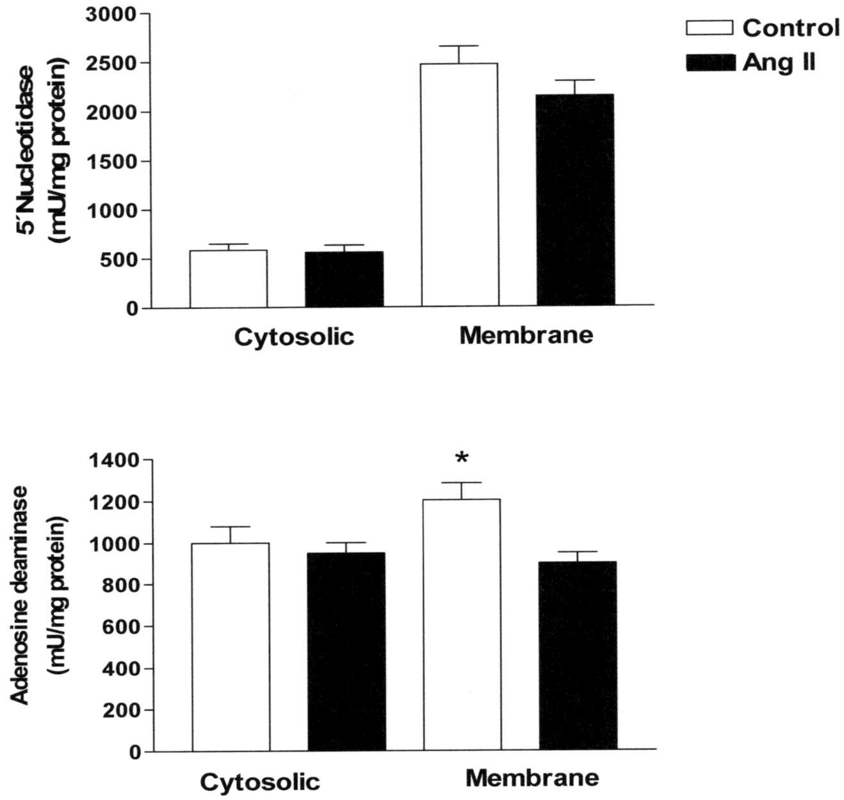

Fig. 5. 5´nucleotidase and adenosine deaminase activities in cytosolic and membrane fractions from control and Ang II treated rats. *$p < 0.05$ vs. cytosolic fraction (modified from Franco et al. 2008).

Furthermore, the adenosine receptor expression was modified in the Ang II hypertensive rat; in this model, it was observed an imbalance between the receptors that mediate vasoconstriction (A1) and vasodilation (A2) that could influence the renal Ang II-mediated vasoconstriction. When adenosine receptors were evaluated, the A1 receptors protein did not change significantly in either the cortex or the medulla, indicating a lack of regulation by the high adenosine concentrations (Franco el al., 2008), which has not been observed with an acute infusion of Ang II; the adaptation of adenosine receptors to chronic exposure to the agonist remains to be determined. In this regard, the A1 receptor require up to 6 days in rat adipocytes for desensitization, (Palmer & Stiles, 1997), and a slight but significant decrease in the high affinity A2a receptor and no change in the low affinity A2b receptors were observed, indicating down regulation of the former (Figure 6).

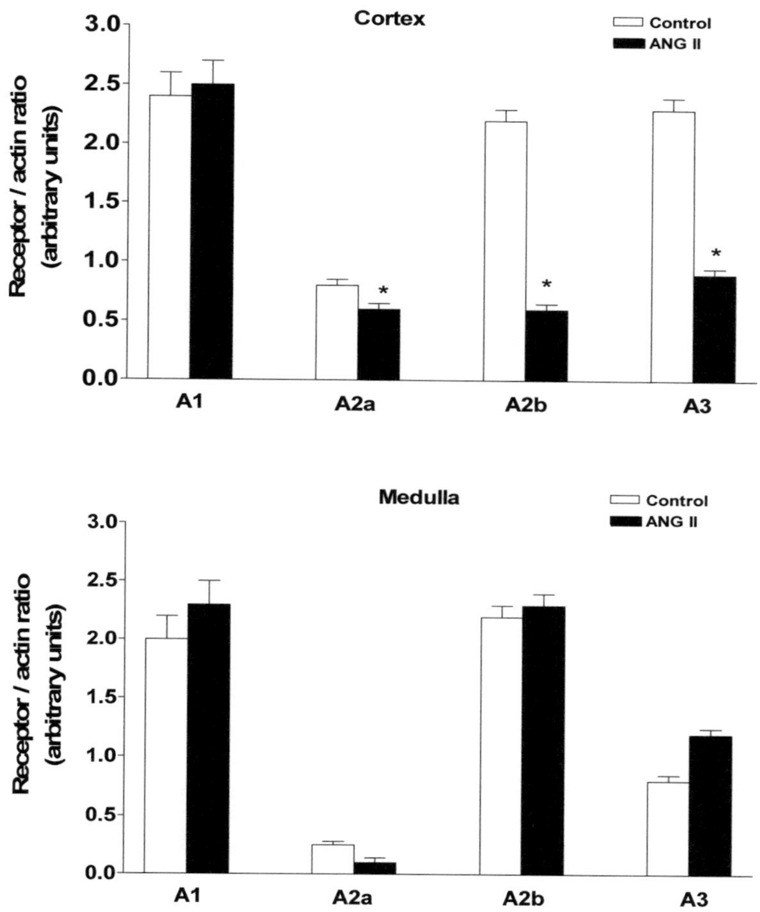

Fig. 6. Adenosine receptor protein expression in renal cortex (top) and medulla (bottom) from control and Ang II treated rats. *$p<0.05$ vs. control rats (modified from Franco et al. 2008).

This finding is in agreement with the fast response of A2a receptors to high levels of adenosine acutely administered (Palmer & Stiles, 1997). Normal expression of A1 receptors population with a decrease in A2a receptors, associated to an elevated concentration of adenosine, may explain synergic effect of adenosine to Ang II-induced renal vasoconstriction (Franco et al., 2001). This notion was further supported by the results obtained in the micropuncture studies; the acute blockade of A1 receptors with the intra-aortic administration of the specific A1 antagonist DPCPX completely reverted the renal vasoconstriction induced by Ang II. These unexpected results clearly demonstrate the great contribution of adenosine in the renal vasoconstriction of the Ang II-infused hypertensive rat. We can attribute the vasodilatory effect of the blocker to an overriding effect of A2 receptors; the reason for this marked vasodilatory response to the specific adenosine A1 antagonist remains to be elucidated.

We also demonstrated an increase in the expression of A3 receptors (Franco et al 2008). In this regard, the physiological effect of A3 receptors in the kidney remains unclear. However, up regulation of these receptors has been associated with deleterious effects in renal function in the renal ischemia-reperfusion model (Lee et al., 2003). In the Ang II-mediated hypertensive model, they could have a similar effect, since ischemia has also been observed (Welch et al., 2005)

4. Participation of ATP to the renal vasoconstriction of the Ang II-infused hypertensive rat

As mentioned above, chronic Ang II infusion lead to a progressive increase in arterial pressure associated with renal vasoconstriction thus maintaining at low levels the renal blood flow and the glomerular filtration rate. Since high arterial pressure result in elevated interstitial levels of ATP in the kidney, which contribute to the autoregulatory-associated responses in microvascular resistances, it is suitable to consider that some of the elevation in vascular resistances observed in Ang II-induced hypertension is modulated by purinergic receptors (Franco et al., 2008). Furthermore, ATP participates in the regulation of vascular resistance and is elevated in Ang II-induced hypertension (Graciano et al., 2008). These observations suggest a modulatory role of ATP in the renal vasoconstriction induced by temporal administration of Ang II. Thus, we explored the possible contribution of ATP

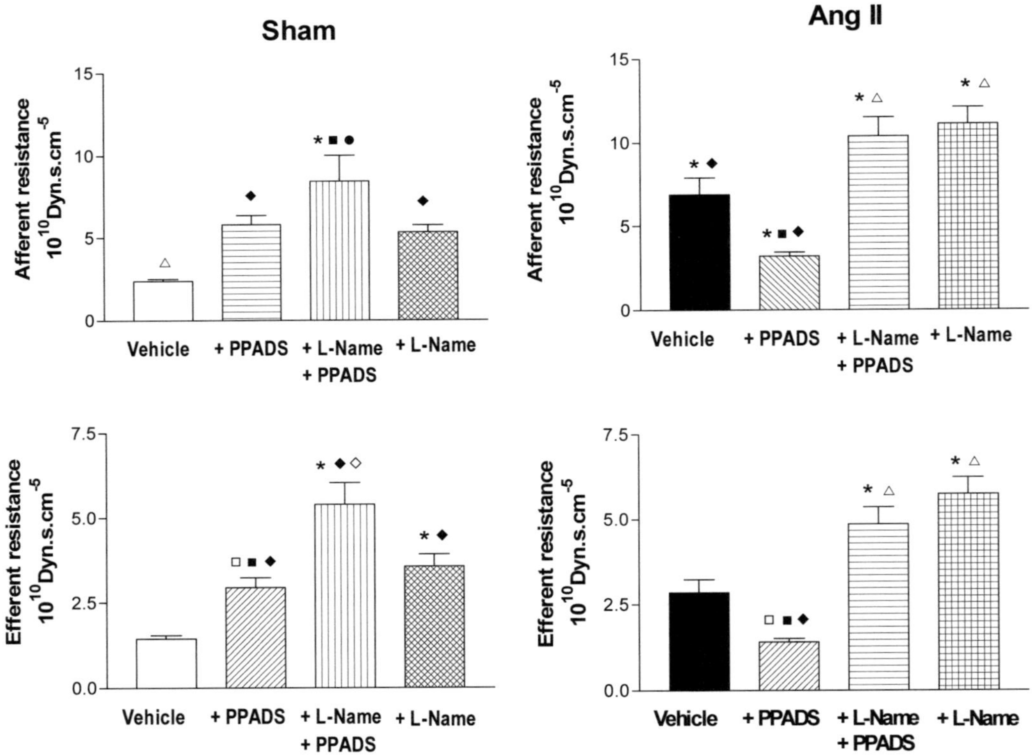

Fig. 7. Afferent and efferent resistances in Sham-control and Ang II groups at baseline, during he administration of PPADS, and the co-administration of L-NAME+PPADS and L-Name alone. * $p<0.001$ vs. Sham-vehicle; △ $p<0.01$ vs. Ang II+vehicle; ◊ $p<0.01$ vs. Sham+L-NAME; ■ $p<0.001$ vs. Ang II+PPADS; ●$p<0.01$ vs. Ang II+PPADS+L-NAME; ◆$p<0.01$ vs. Ang II+L-NAME (modified from Franco et al. 2011)

purinergic receptors in the renal hemodynamics and glomerular alterations observed in the Ang II-mediated hypertension in rats. Ang II-induced renal vasoconstriction, an the acute administration of PPADS, (a P2X and P2Y antagonist), reduced afferent and efferent resistances, restoring glomerular blood flow and single nephron glomerular filtration rate (Figures 7 and 8).

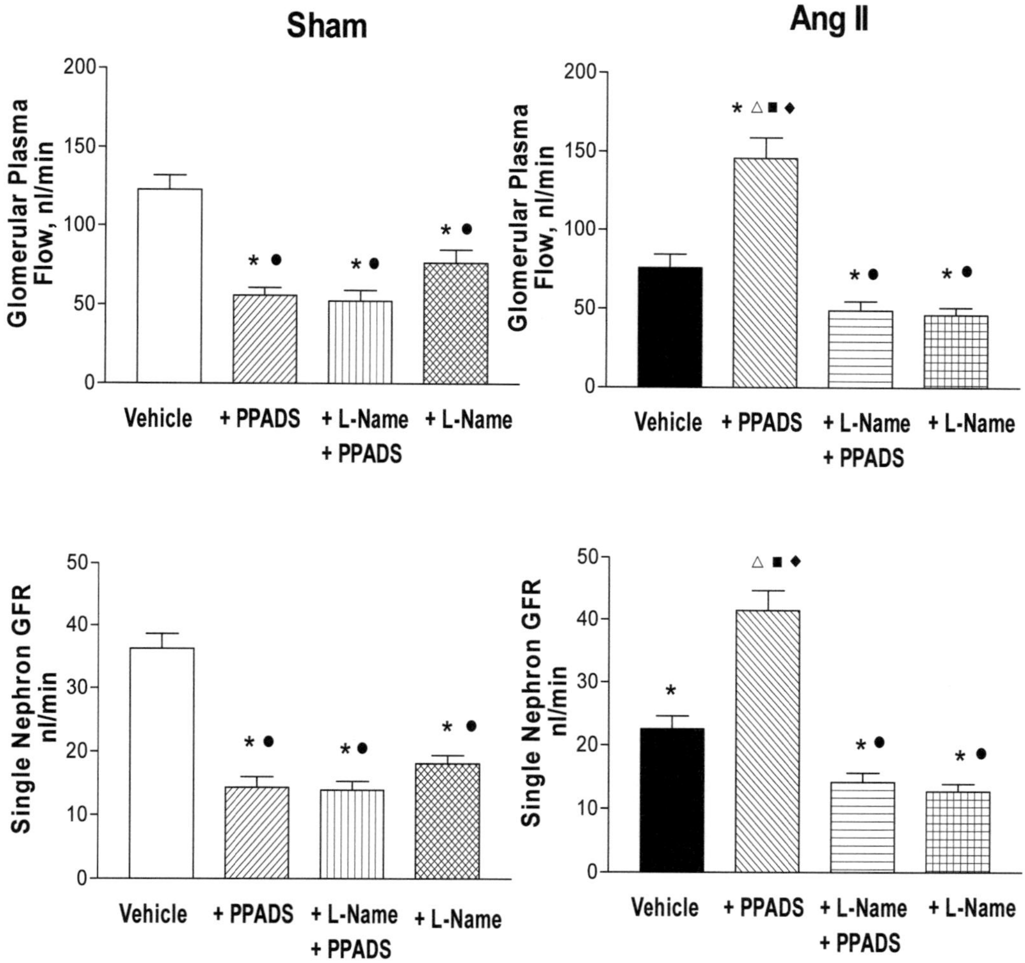

Fig. 8. Glomerular plasma flow and single nephron GFR, in Sham-control and Ang II groups at baseline, during the administration of PPADS, and the co-administration of L-NAME+PPADS and L-NAME alone. *p<0.001 vs. Sham-vehicle; △ p< 0.01 vs. Ang II+vehicle; Sham+PPADS; ■ p<0.001 vs. Ang II+PPADS; ● p<0.01 vs. Ang II+PPADS+L-NAME (modified from Franco et al. 2011).

These changes in glomerular hemodynamics cannot be attributed to modifications in blood pressure, since PPADS did not ameliorate the elevated blood pressure neither in the Ang II group, nor the Sham group. These findings suggest an important contribution of ATP in mediating the renal vasoconstriction via activation of P2 purinergic receptors. Interestingly, P2X and P2Y receptors are expressed primarily in afferent but not in efferent arterioles; therefore, the effects of PPADS on efferent arterioles suggest the presence of additional systems that become activated after purinergic blockade in the Ang II-infused rats (Chan et al., 1998; Ichihara et al., 1998; Lambrecht, 2000; Lewis & Evans, 2001; Turner et al., 2003). In addition, PX1 and P2Y1 receptors expression in the cortex of Ang II rats was significantly higher on the immunohistochemical studies (Figure 9).

Several mechanisms may be involved in the renal vasodilation induced by PPADS; P2X1 receptors were upregulated in the cortical tissue of the Ang II group. Therefore, the increased number of these receptors may have been exerting a direct effect on the vascular smooth muscle to increase renal vascular resistance, and their blockade induces vasodilation. It is possible that P2X1 blockade unmask the influence of P2Y receptors as P2y2, P2y4, P2Y6 and P2Y12, which are not blocked by PPADS (Lambrecht, 2000), and those P2Y receptors may exert vasodilatory effects on the smooth muscle cells via release of NO by the endothelial cells, thus helping to explain the decrease in efferent resistance (Jackson, et al, 2007) as shown in figure 7 (Franco, 2008), in which the blockade of NO with L-NAME prevents the vasodilator effect of PPADS (Lambrecht, 1996; Lambrecht, 2000). In this regard, P2X4 receptors have been described in endothelial cells, and they induce NO release (Burnstock, 2006; Jones et al., 2000). However, the activation of P2X1 receptors also stimulates p-450 pathway and induces production of the vasoconstrictor HETE (Zhao et al, 2001) and this mechanism may be blocked by PPADS, resulting in vasodilation. In addition, PPADS increased NO productions, which also inhibit HETE synthesis (Oyecan & McGiff, 2002); thus, both mechanisms (which occurred simultaneously) may explain the vasodilation observed in theAng II rats.

Since purinergic blockade may modify the release of NO production, further studies were performed to investigate the role of NO in the response to PPADS. Importantly, using the urinary excretion of nitrites (UNO_2^-/NO_3^-) as a marker of NO activity, we found that it was low in the Ang II-infused rats compared with Sham rats at baseline, but increased greatly with the infusion of PPADS (Franco et al 2011). These results suggesting that NO produced by the endothelial cells was directly stimulated by PPADS, or maybe through an effect on P2Y or P2X receptors not blocked by PPADS to release NO and elicit vasodilation (Figure 10).

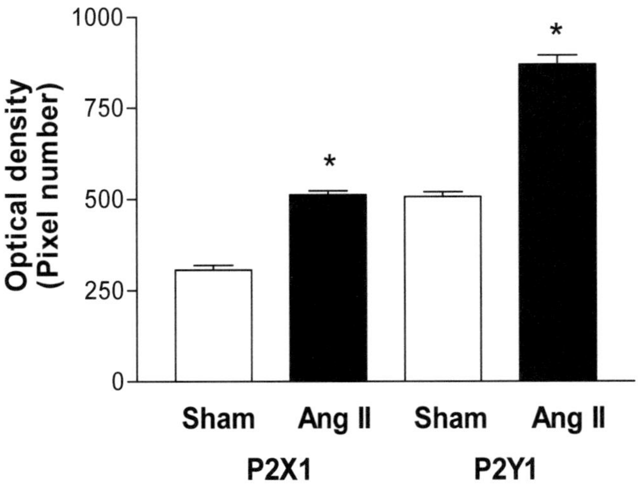

Fig. 9. P2X1 and P2Y1 immunostaining evaluated by morphometric analysis (expressed as pixel number) in the cortex of Sham-control and Ang II treated rats.* p<0.0001 vs. Sham (modified from Franco et al. 2011)

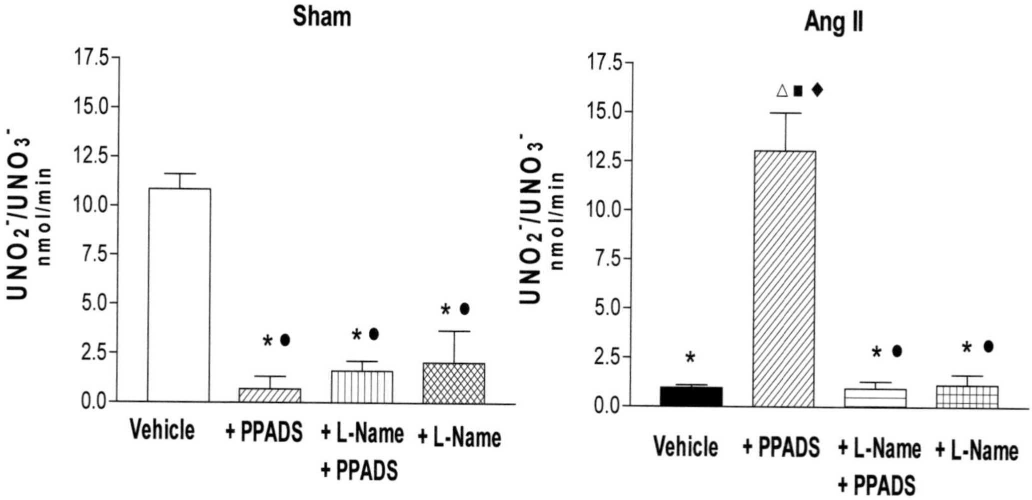

Fig. 10. Urinary excretion of nitrites/ nitrates (UNO_2^-/NO_3^-) from Sham-control and Ang II groups at baseline, during PPADS and coadministration of L-NAME+PPADS, and L-NAME alone. * $p<0.001$ vs. Sham-vehicle; △ $p< 0.01$ vs.Ang II+ vehicle; • $p<0.001$ vsAng II+PPADS; ■ $p<0.001$ vs. Ang II+L-NAME +PPADS; ♦ $p<0.01$ vs. Ang II+L-NAME (modified from Franco et al. 2011)

This finding was supported by the results observed upon co-administration of PPADS and L-NAME, which returned NO_2^-/NO_3^- urinary levels to those found al baseline, thus suggesting the existence of NO-mediated dilation in the PPADS group (Franco et al. 2011). in our study this possibility is further supported by the fact that blockade of NO with L-NAME alone elicited effects similar to those obtained with PPADS+L-NAME (Franco et al. 2011). In this regard, it is recognized that activation of P2Y receptors induces release of ATP by shear stress in the endothelial cells, through an increase on intracellular calcium, which activates NOS and NO production in the endothelium (Buvinic et al., 2002).

In a study, a low NO can explain the efferent vasoconstriction, which returned to near-normal values when NO increased in response to PPADS (Inscho et al., 1992). In addition, although PPADS is a non-selective P2 receptor antagonist, it is very specific for purinergic receptors (Windscheif et al., 1994), it also blocks ecto-ATPasas (Chen et al., 1996; Lambrecht, 2000) and it may not block P2Y2 and P2Y12 receptors (Lambrecht, 1996; Lambrecht, 2000; Rost et al., 2002). It should be noticed that in the Sham rats PPADS induced a paradoxical renal vasoconstriction, as manifested by an increase in afferent and efferent resistance, and a reduction in glomerular blood flow, SNGFR and Kf. These responses indicate that the effects of P2 receptors in normal control rats are primarily vasodilator and can be attributed to the existence of a P2 receptor population in the endothelium, linked to NO release in the kidneys of Sham rats. Thus, it is possible that the renal vasoconstriction in this group may be due to blockade of P2Y1 or P2X4 receptors on the endothelial cells (Chen et al., 1996; Boyer et al., 1994; Curchill & Ellis, 1993). As above-mentioned, it has been demonstrated that P2X4 receptors are located in the endothelial cells and are linked to NO release, leading to vasodilation in dome vessels (Burnstock, 2006; Lewis, 2001; Yamamoto, 2006). Thus the blockade of P2X4 receptors by high concentrations of PPADS would decrease NO production and induce vasoconstriction (Jones et al. 2000) and could explain the findings that the efferent as well the afferent arteriolar resistances were reduced. Under these conditions, the co-administration of PPADS with L-NAME was not expected to have a much greater additional effect, which was the case in the Sham rats. However, we cannot rule out that, in the presence of NO blockade the effect of endogenous vasoconstrictor mediators could be enhanced and alter renal function. It is recognized that the renal vasoconstriction observed in the Sham rats with PPADS (Franco et al. 2011) was not observed by Tanaka el al (Takenaka et al., 2008) or Osmond and Inscho (Osmond & Inscho, 2010); these authors used an intravenous bolus, each 20 min with a lower dose than ours. Under those conditions, lower concentrations of PPADS possible reach the kidney; however the dose used in those studies (Osmond & Inscho, 2010) were sufficient to block P2 receptors as evidenced by the blockade of the vasoconstrictor response to α,βmethylene ATP; thus an explanation for the divergent effects of PPADS in Sham rats remains to be elucidated.

We also observed that sodium excretion was increased by PPADS in both Sham and Ang II-infused rats, suggesting that the increase P2 receptor activity inhibits tubular reabsorption. These data are similar to those found in rats receiving a low salt diet (Dobrowolski et al., 2007). The co-administration of L-NAME further increases sodium elimination, but inhibits NO excretion; however, the increase in sodium excretion induced by L-NAME alone was lower, than the Ang II group indicating that NO partially mediated the increase in sodium excretion. It should be mentioned, that the increase in sodium excretion, mainly in the Ang II group, was associated with a marked decrease in the urinary excretion of NO_2^-/NO_3^- indicating that the NO_2^-/NO_3^- is a specific marker of renal NO production in this model and it is not the result of nonspecific increased urinary sodium excretion.

These results indicate that temporal Ang II infusion up-regulates P2X1 receptors, which may contribute to increases the renal cortical vascular resistance observed in the Ang II-dependent hypertension. The results also indicate that in Ang II-infused rats PPADS may elicit a marked stimulation of NO, which may also contribute the reduced afferent and efferent arteriolar resistance.

5. Conclusions

The renal vasoconstriction induced by chronic administration of angiotensin II is complex, since several vasoactive compounds contribute to the abnormalities induced by the peptide in the renal glomerular hemodynamics. The results obtained in our studies indicate that the temporal infusion of Ang II, produces elevation of renal tissue content and interstitial concentration of adenosine which contributes to the renal vasoconstriction observed in this model. Our studies suggest that the mechanism by which Ang II increases adenosine production is through the extracellular nucleotide degradation of ATP, as well as a decrease of ecto-ADA, that impairs adenosine degradation; the elevated adenosine thus induce an imbalance en A1 and A2 receptors. Since the ATP seems to be related in a very importantly manner with the results obtained in our first study, we further investigated the participation of ATP in the renal vasoconstriction observed during the chronic infusion of angiotensin II. We found that Ang II regulates P2X1 receptors, and contributes to increase the renal vascular resistance observed in the ANG II-dependent hypertension. Under these conditions PPADS, a non selective ATP receptors blocker (P2X and P2Y receptors) elicit a marked stimulation of NO production which contributes to reduce afferent and efferent arteriolar resistances, normalizes the glomerular blood flow and the ultrafiltration coefficient, resulting in a normalization of the single glomerular filtration rate and renal function return to normal values. Thus, elevation of ATP and adenosine contributes to the alteration in renal hemodynamics in the Ang II-induced hypertension.

6. Acknowledgment

This work was supported by grant number 79661 from Conacyt to M. Franco.

7. References

Arendshorst WJ.; Brännstrom, K.; Ruan X. (1999). Actions of Angiotensin II on the Renal Microvasculature. *Journal of the American Society of Nephrology*, Vol.10, No. Suppl.1, (January 1999), pp. S149-S161, ISSN 1533-3450

Blantz, RC.; Konnen, KS.; Tucker BJ. (1976). Angiotensin II Effects upon the Glomerular Microcirculation and Ultrafiltration Coefficient of the Rat. *Journal of Clinical Investigation*, Vol.57, No.2, (February 1976) pp. 419-434, ISSN 0021-9738

Boyer, JL.; Zohn, IE.; Jacobson , KA.; Harden, TK. (1994). Differential Effects of P2-Purinoceptor Antagonist nn Phospholipase C and Adenyl Cycles Coupled P2Y-Purinoceptors. *British Journal of Pharmacology*, Vol.113, No.2, (October 1994), pp. 614-620, ISSN 1476-5381

Burnstock, G. (2007). Purine and Pyrimidin Receptors. Cellular and Molecular Life Sciences, Vol. 64, No 12 (Jun 2007), pp. 1471-1483, ISSN0916-0636

Burnstock, G. (2006). Purinergic Signaling. *British Journal of Pharmacology*, Vol.147, No.S1, (January 2006), pp. S172-S181, ISSN 1476-5381

Burnstock, G. (2006). Vessel Tone and Remodeling. *Nature Medicine*, Vol.12, No.1, (January 2006), pp. 16-17, ISSN 1078-1989

Buvinic, S.; Briones, R; Huidoro-Toro JP. (2002.) P2Y(1) and P2Y(2) Receptors are Coupled to the NO/cGMP Pathway to Vasodilate the Rat Arterial Mesenterial Bed. *British Journal of Pharmacology*, Vol.136, No.6, (July 2002), pp. 847-856, ISSN 1476-5381

Chan, CM.; Unwin, RJ.; Bardini, M.; Oglesby, IB.; Ford, AP.; Townsend-Nicholson , A.; Burnstock G. (1998). Localization of P2X1 Purinoceptors by Autoradiography and Immunohistochemistry in Rat Kidneys. *American Journal of Physiology, Renal Physiology*, Vol.274, No.4, (April 1998), pp. F799-F804, ISSN 0363-6127

Chen, BC.; Lee, CM.; Lin, WW. (1996). Inhibition of Ecto-ATPase by PPADS, Suramin and Reactive Blue in Endothelial Cells, C6 Glioma Cells and RAW 264.7 Macrophages. *British Journal of Pharmacology*, Vol.110, No.8, (December 1996), pp. 1628-1634, ISSN 1476-5381

Churchill, PC.; Ellis, VR. (1993). Pharmacological Characterization of the Renovascular Purinergic P2 Receptors. *Journal of Pharmacology and Experimental Therapeutics*, Vol.265, No.1, (April 1993), pp. 334-338, ISSN 0022-3565

Dietrich, HH.; Endlich, K.; Parekh, N.; Steinhousen M. (2000). Red Blood Cell Regulation of Microvascuar Tone Through Adenosine Triphosphate. *American Journal of Physiology, Heart Circulatory Physiology*, Vol. 278, No.4, (April 2000), pp. H1294-H1298, ISSN 0363-6135

Dobrowolski, L.; Walkowska, A; Kompanowska-Jezierska, E.; Kuczeriszka, M.; Sadowsky J. (2007). Effects of ATP on Rat Renal Haemodynamics and Excretion: Role of Sodium

Intake, Nitric Oxide and Cytochrome P 450. *Acta Physiologica*, Vol.189, No.1, (January 2007), pp. 77-85, ISSN 17481716

Franco, M.; Navar, LG.; Bell PD. (1989). Effect of Adenosine 1 Analogue on Tubuloglomerular Feedack Mechanism. *American Journal of Physiology, Renal Electrolite Physiology*, Vol.257, No.2, (August 1989), pp. F231-F296, ISSN 0363-6127

Franco, M.; Bobadilla, NA.; Suárez, J.; Tapia E.; Sánchez, L.; Herrera-Acosta J. (1996). Participation of Adenosine in the Renal Hemodynamic Abnormalities of Hypothyroidism. *American Journal of Physiology, Renal, Fluid Electrolyte Physiology*, Vol.270, No.2, (February 1996), pp. F 254-F262, ISSN 0363-6127

Franco, M.; Tapia, E.; Santamaría, J.; Zafra, I.; García-Torres, R.; Gordon, KL.; Pons, H.; Rodríguez-Iturbe, B.; Johnson, JR.; Herrera-Acosta J. (2001). Renal Cortical Vasoconstriction Contributes to the Development of Salt Sensitive Hypertension after Angiotensin II Exposure. *Journal of the American Society of Nephrology*, Vol.10, No.11,(November 2001), pp. 2263-2271, ISSN:1533-3450

Franco, M., Martínez, F.; Rodríguez-Iturbe, B.; Johnson, RJ.; Santamaría J.; Montoya A.; Nepomuceno, T.; Bautista, R.; Tapia E.; Herrera-Acosta J. Angiotensin II, Interstitial Inflammation and the Pathogenesis of Salt-Sensitive Hypertension. (2006). *American Journal of Physiology, Renal Physiology*, Vol.291, No.6, (December 2006), pp. F1281-F1287, ISSN 0363-6127

Franco, M.; Bautista, R.; Pérez-Méndez, O.; González, L.; Pacheco, U.; Sánchez-Lozada, LG.; Tapia, E.; Moreal, R.; Martínez, F. (2008). Renal Interstitial adenosine is increased in angiotensin II-induced hypertensive rats. *American Journal of Physiology,Renal Physiology*, Vol. 294, No. 1, (January 2008), pp. F84-F92, ISSN 0363-6127

Franco, M.; Bautista, R.; Tapia, E.; Soto, V.; Santamaría, J.; Osorio, H.; Pacheco, U.; Sánchez-Lozada, LG.; Kobori, H.; Navar, LG. F. (2011). Contribution of renal purinergic receptors to renal vasoconstriction in angiotensin II-induced hypertensive rats. *American Journal of Physiology,Renal Physiology*, Vol. 300, No. 6, (June 2011), pp. F1301-1309, ISSN 0363-6127

Graciano, ML.; Nishiyama, A.; Jackson, K.; Seth, DM.; Ortiz, RM.; Prieto-Carrasquero, M.; Kobori, H.; Navar LG. (2008). Purinergic Receptors Contribute to Early Mesangial Transformation and Renal Vessel Hypertrophy during Angiotensin II-Induced Hypertension. *American Journal of Physiology, Renal Physiology*, Vol.294, No.1, (January 2008), pp. F161-F169, ISSN 0363-6127

Gordon , EL.; Pearson, DJ.; Dickinson, ES.; Moreau, D.; Sakey, LL. (1989). The Hydrolysis of Extracellular Adenine Nucleotides by Arterial Smooth Muscle Cells. Regulation of Adenosine Production at the Cell Surface. *Journal of Biological Chemistry*, Vol.264, No.32, (November 1989), pp. 18986-18992, ISSN 0021-9258

Guang, Z.; Osmond, DA.; Inscho, EW. (2007). Purinoceptors in the Kidney. *Experimental Biology and Medicine*. Vol. 232, No. 6, (June 2007), pp. 715-726, ISSN 065-2598

Hall, JE.; Granger, JP. (1986). Adenosine Alters Glomerular Filtration Control by Angiotensin II. *American Journal of Physiology, Renal Fluid, Electrolyte Physiology*, Vol.250, No.5, (May 1986), pp. F917-F923, ISSN 0363-6127

Hall, JE.; Granger, JP.; Hester RL. (1985). Interaction Between Adenosine and Angiotensin II in Controlling Glomerular Filtration. *American Journal of Physiology, Renal Fluid, electrolyte Physiology*, Vol.248, No.3, (March 1986), pp. F340-F346, ISSN 0363-6127

Hansen, PB.; Hashimoto, S.; Briggs, J.; Schnermann J. (2003). Attenuated Renovascular Constrictor Responses to Angiotensin II in Adenosine 1 Receptor Knockout Mice. *American Journal of Physiology, Regulatory Integrative comprehensive Physiology,* Vol.285, No.1, (July, 2003), pp. R44-R49, ISSN 0363-6119

Ichicara, A.; Iming, JD.; Inscho, EW.; Navar LG. (1998). Interactive Nitric Oxide-Angiotensin II Influences on Renal Microcirculation in Angiotensin II Induced Hypertension. *Hypertension,* Vol.31, No.6, (June 1998), pp. 1255-1260, ISSN 0194-911X

Inscho, EW. (2009). ATP, P2 Receptors and the Renal Microcirculation. *Purinergic signaling,* Vol.5, No.4, (Month 2009), pp. 447-460, ISSN1573-9538

Inscho, EW. (2001). P2 Receptors in the Regulation of Renal Microvascular Function. *American Journal of Physiology , Renal Physiology,* Vol.280, No.6, (June 2001), pp. F927-F944, ISSN 0363-6127

Inscho, EW.; Cook, AK.; Navar LG. (1996). Pressure-mediated Vasoconstriction of Juxtamedullary Afferent Arterioles Involves P2-purinoceptors Activation. *American Journal of Physiology, Renal Physiogy,* Vol.271, No.5, Pte 2, (November 1996), pp. F1077-F1085, ISSN 0363-6127

Inscho, EW.; Ohichi, K.; Cook, AK.; Belott, TP.; Navar LG. (1995). Calcium Activation Mechanisms in the Renal Microvascular Response to Extracellular ATP. *American Journal of Physiology, Renal Physiology,* Vol.268 No.5, (May 1995), pp. F876-F884, ISSN 0363-6127

Inscho, EW.; Mitchell, KD; Navar LG. (1994). Extracellular ATP in the Regulation of Renal Microvascular Function. *Faseb Journal,* Vol.8, No.3, (March 1 1994), pp. 319-328, ISSN 0892-6638

Inscho, EW.; Ohishi, K.; Navar, LG. (1992). Effects of ATP on Pre and Post-glomerular Juxtamedullary Microvasculature. *American journal of Physiology, Renal Fluid, Electrolite Physiology,* Vol.263, No.5, (November 1992), pp. F8856-F893, ISSN 0363-6127.

Jackson, EK.; Dubey, RK. (2001). Role of Extracellular c-AMP-Adenosine Pathway in Renal Physiology. *American journal of Physiology, Renal Physiology,* Vol.281, No.4, (October 2001), pp. F597-F612, ISSN 0363-6127

Jackson, EK.; Mi, Z.; Dubey RK. (2007). The Extracellular cAMP-Adenosine Pathway Significantly Contributes to the In Vivo Production of Adenosine. *Journal of Pharmacology and Experimental Therapeutics,* Vol.321, No.1, (January 2007), pp. 117-123, ISSN 0022-3565

Jones, CA.; Chessel, IP; Simon, J.; Barnard EA.; Miller, KJ.; Michel, AD.; Humphrey, PPA. (2000). Functional Characterization of the P2X4 Receptor Orthologues. *British Journal of Pharmacology,* Vol.129, No.2, (January 2000), pp. 388-394, ISSN 1476-5381

Johnson, RJ.; Alpers CE.; Yoshimura, A.; Lombardi, D.; Pritzl P.; Floege, J.; Schwartz SM. (1992). Renal Injury from Angiotensin II-Mediated Hypertension. *Hypertension,* Vol.19, No.5 (May 1992), pp. 464-474, ISSN 0194-911X

Lai, EY.; Fähling, M.; Ma, Z.; Källskog,O.; Persson, PB.; Patzak, A.; Persson, AE.; Hulström, M. (2009). Norepinephrine Increases Calcium Sensitivity of Mouse Afferent Arteriole, Thereby Enhancing Angiotensin II-Mediated Vasoconstriction. *Kidney International,* Vol.76, No.9, (November 2009), pp. 953-959, ISSN 0085-2538

Lambrecht, G. (1996) Design and Pharmacology of Selective P2-Purinoceptors Antagonists. *Journal of Autonomic Pharmacology,* Vol.16, No.6, (December 1996), pp. 953-959, ISSN 1474-8673

Lambrecht, G. (2000). Agonists and Antagonists Acting at P2X Receptors: Selectivity Profiles and Functional Implications. *Naunyn-Schmiedeberg´s Archives of Pharmacology*, Vol.362, No.4-5, (November 2000), pp. 340-350, ISSN 0028-1298

Lee, HT.; Ota-Setlik, A.; Xu, H.; Dágati, VD.; Jacobson, MA.; Emala, CW. A3 Adenosine Receptor Knockout Mice are Protected Against Ischemia- and Myoglobinuria-Induced Renal Failure. (2003). *American Journal of Physiology, Renal Physiology*, Vol.284, No.2, (February 2003), pp F287-F273, ISSN 0363-6127

Lewis, CJ.; Evans RJ. (2001). Receptor Immunoreactivity in Different Arteries from the Femoral, Pulmonary, Coronary and Renal Circulations. *Journal of Vascular Research*, Vol.38, No.4, (July-August 2001), pp. 332-340, ISSN 0363-6127

Lombardi, D.; Gordon, Kl.; Polinski, P.; Suga, S.; Schwartz, SM.; Johnson RJ. (1999). Salt Sensitive Hypertension Develops after Short Term Exposure to Angiotensin II. *Hypertension*, Vol.33, No.4, (April 1999), pp. 1013-1019, ISSN 0194-911X

Mitchell, KD. and Navar, LG. (1993). Modulation of Tubuloglomerular Feedback Responsiveness by Extracelular ATP. *American Journal of Physiology, Renal Fluid, Electrolyte Physiology*, Vol.264, No.3, (March 1993), pp. F458-F466, ISSN 0363-6127

Navar, LG.; Harrison-Bernard, LM.; Nishiyama, A.; Kobori H. (2002). Regulation of Intrarenal Angiotensin II in Hypertension. *Hypertension*, Vol.39, Vol.2, (February 2002), pp. 316-322, ISSN 0194-911X

Navar, LG. (1998). Integrating Multiple Paracrine Regulators on Renal Microvascular Dynamics. *American Journal of Physiology, Renal Physiology*, Vol.274. No.3, (March 1998), pp F433-F444, ISSN 0363-6127

Nishiyama, A.; Kimura, S.; He, H.; Miura, K.;Rahman, M.; Fujisawa, Y.; Fukui Abe, YT. (2001). Renal Interstitial Adenosine Metabolism During Ischemia in Dogs. *American journal of Physiology, Renal Physiology*, Vol.280, No.2, (February 2001), pp. F231-F238, ISSN 0363-6127

Osmond, DA.; Inscho, EW. (2010). P2X1 Receptor Blockade Inhibits Whole Kidney Autoregulation of Renal Blood Flow In Vivo. *American Journal of Physiology, Renal Physiology*, Vol.298, No.6, (June 2010), pp.F1360-F1368, ISSN 0363-6127

Osswald, H. (1984). The Role of Adenosine in the Regulation of Glomerular Filtration Rate and Renin Secretion. *Trends in Pharmacologial Sciences,* Vol. 5, pp. 94-97, ISSN 0165-6547

Oyecan, AO.; McGiff, JC. (1998). Functional Response of the Rat Kidney to Inhibition of Nitric Oxide Synthesis: Role of Cytochrome P450-Derived Arachidonate Metabolites. *British Journal of Pharmacology*, Vol.125, No.5, (November 1998), pp. 1065-1073, ISSN 1476-5381

Ozawa, Y.; Kobori, H.; Suzaki, Y.; Navar LG. (2007). Sustained Renal Interstitial Macrophague Infiltration Following Chronic Angiotensin II Infusions. *American Journal of Physiology, Renal Physiology*, Vol.292, No.1, (January 2007) pp. F330-F339, ISSN 0363-6127

Palmer, TM.; Stiles GL. (1997) Structure-Function Analysis of Inhibitory Adenosine Receptor Regulation. *Neuropharmacology*,Vol.36, No.9,(September 1997), pp. 1141-1147, ISSN 0028-3908

Rodriguez-Iturbe, B.; Pons, H.; Herrera-Acosta, J. ,Johnson RJ. (2001). Role of Immunocompetent Cells in Non Immune Renal Disease. *Kidney International*, Vol.59, No.5, (May 2001), pp.1626-1640, ISSN 0085-2538

Rost, S.; Daniel, C.; Schultze-Lohoff, E.; Bäumert, HG.; Lambreacht, G.; Hugo, C. (2002). P2 Antagonist PPADS Inhibits Mesangial Cell Proliferation in Experimental Mesangial Proliferative Glomerulonephritis. *Kidney International,* Vol.62, No.5, (November 2002), pp. 1659-1671, ISSN 0085-2538

Ruiz-Ortega, M.; Ruperez, M.; Esteban, V.; Egido, J. (2003). Molecular Mechanisms of Angiotensin II-Induced Vascular Injury. *Current Hypertension Reports,* Vol.5, No.1 (February 2003, pp. 73-79, ISSN 1522-6417

Sasser, JM.; Pollock, JS.; Pollock, DM. (2002). Renal Endothelin on Chronic Angiotensin II Hypertension. *American Journal of Physiology, Regulatory Integrative Comprehensive Physiology,* Vol.283, No.1, (July 2002), pp. R243-R248, ISSN 0363-6119

Schnermann, J.; Levine, DZ. (2003). Paracrine Factors in the Tubuloglomerular Feedback: Adenosine, ATP, and Nitric Oxide. *Annual Review of Physiology,* Vol.65, No.1, (March 2003), pp. 501-529, ISSN 0066-4278

Shao, W.; Seth, DM.; Navar LG. (2009). Augmentation of Endogenous Intrarenal Angiotensin II Levels in Val5-AngII-Infused Rats. *American Journal of Physiology, Renal Physiology,* Vol.296, No.5, (May 2009), pp. F1067-F1071, ISSN 0363-6127

Suzuki, Y.; Ruiz-Ortega, M.; Gomez-Guerrero C.; Tomino, Y.; Egido J. (2003).Inflammation and Angiotensin II. *International Journal of Biochemistry & cell Biology,* Vol.35, No.6, (June 2003), pp. 881-900, ISSN 1357-2725

Takenaka, T.; Inoue T, Kanno, Y.; Okada, H.; Hill, CE.; Suzuki H. (2008). Connexins 37 and 40 Transduce Purinergic Signals Mediating Renal Autoregulation. *American Journal of Physiology, Regulative and Comprehensive Physiology,* Vol.294, No.1, (January 2008), pp. R1-R11, ISSN 0363-6119

Turner, CM.; Vonend, O.; Chan, C.; Burnstock, G., Unwin, RJ. (2003). The Pattern of Distribution of Selected ATP-Sensitive P2 Receptor Subtypes in Normal Rat Kidney: An Immunohistological Study. *Cells Tissues Organs,* Vol.175, No.2, (September 2003), pp. 105-117, ISSN 1422-6405

Weihprecht, H.; Lorenz, JN.; Briggs, JP.; Schnermann, J. (1994).Synergistic Effects of Angiotensin and Adenosine in the Renal Microvasculature. *American Journal of Physiology, Renal Electrolyte Physiology,* Vol.266, No.2, (February 1994), pp. F227-F239, ISSN 0363-6127

Windscheif, U.; Ralevic, V.; Bäumert, HG.; Mutscler, E.; Lambrecht, G.; Burnstock, G. (1994). Vasoconstrictor and Vasodilator Responses to Various Agonists and Antagonist in the Rat Perfused Mesenteric Arterial Bed: Selective Inhibition by PPADS of Contraction Mediated Via P2X-Purinoceptors. *British Journal of Pharmacology,* Vol.113, No.3, (November 1994), pp. 1015-1021, ISSN 1476-5381.

Welch, WJ.; Blau, J.; Xie, H.; Chabrashvili, T.; Wilcox, CS. (2005). Angiotensin-induced defects in renal oxygenation: role of oxidative stress. *American Journal of Physiology, Heart Circulatory Physiology,* Vol. 288, No. 1, (January 2005), pp. H22-H28, ISSN 0363-6135

Wihlborg, AK.; Malmsjö, M.; Eyjolfsson, A.; Gustafsson, R.; Jacobson, K.; Erlinge, D.(2003). Extracellular Nucleotides Induce Vasodilatation in Human Arteries Via Prostaglandins, Nitric Oxide and Endothelium-Derived Hyperpolarizing Factor. *British Journal of Pharmacology,* Vol.138, No.8, (April 2003), pp. 1451-1458, ISSN 1476-5381

Yamamoto, K.; Sokabe, T.; Matsumoto, T.; Yoshimura K, Shibata, M.; Ohura Fukuda, TN.; Sato, T.; Sekine, K.; Kato, S.; Issiki M.; Fujita, T.; Kobayashi, M.; Kawamura, K.; Masuda, H.; Kamiya, A.; Ando, J. (2006). Impaired Flow-Dependent Control of Vascular Tone and Remodeling in P2x4-Deficient Mice. *Nature Medicine*, Vol.12, No.1,(January 2006), pp. 133-137, ISSN 1978-8956

Zhao, X.; Inscho, EW.; Bondlela, M.; Falk, JR.; Iming J. (2001). The CYP450 Hydroxylase Pathway Contributes to P2X Receptor-Mediated Afferent Arteriolar Vasoconstriction. *American Journal of Physiology, Heart Circulatory Physiology*, Vol.281, No.5, (November 2001), pp. H2089-H2096, ISSN 0363-6135

Zou, L-X.;Hymel, A.;Imig, JD.; Navar LG. (1996). Renal Accumulation of Circulating Angiotensin II in AngiotensinII-Infused Rats. *Hypertension*, Vol.27, No.3, (March 1996), pp. 658-662, ISSN 0194-911X

6

Carnosine and Its Role on the Erythrocyte Rheology

A. Seda Artis[1] and Sami Aydogan[2]
[1]*Physiology Department, Medical Faculty, Istanbul Medeniyet University*
[2]*Physiology Department, Medical Faculty, Erciyes University*
Turkey

1. Introduction

Erythrocytes are the most abundant cells (around 5 million/mm^3) in the body. The main function of these specialized cells is transport of oxygen (O_2) and mediation of carbondioxide (CO_2) production (Volpe, 1993). Mature erythrocytes have no capacity for cell division, protein synthesis, and mitochondrial-based oxidative reactions (Bunn, 1991; Benz, 2010). The erythrocyte possesses more membrane surface area than is needed to encase the volume of its cytoplasm. This allows for biconcave disc geometry. This shape can be stretched, twisted, distended, and compressed without permanent damage (Benz, 2010).

Erythrocytes are a highly specialized O_2 carrier system in the body. More than 95% of cytoplasmic protein is hemoglobin (Telen & Kaufman, 1999). Hemoglobin is the protein responsible for the oxygen-carrying capacity of erythrocytes. It provides the binding to O_2 to heme, while keeping iron in the +2 oxidation state to assure the reversibility of this binding. Hemoglobin also facilitates exchange of CO_2 (Nohl & Stolze, 1998; Telen & Kaufman, 1999). Under normal conditions, 95% of hemoglobin is saturated with oxygen in the lungs, whereas under physiologic conditions in peripheral blood stream only 25% of oxygenated hemoglobin becomes deoxygenated. Thus, the major fraction of oxygen bound to hemoglobin is recirculated with venous blood. The use of this fraction has been suggested for the treatment of oxygen deficiency. 2,3-Diphosphoglycerate (2,3-DPG) is a natural effector of hemoglobin. The binding affinity of hemoglobin for oxygen changes reversibly with the concentration of 2,3-DPG in the intracellular compartment. This compensates for changes in the oxygen pressure outside of the body, as the affinity of 2,3-DPG to oxygen is much higher than that of hemoglobin (Guyton & Hall, 2000). The oxygen transport function of erythrocytes depends on the membrane being deformable and the components of the membrane play important roles in this function.

The erythrocyte membrane is composed of proteins (52% in weight), lipids (40%), and carbohydrates (8%). Membrane elasticity depends on the structural interactions between the outer plasma membrane and the underlying protein skeleton (Desouky, 2009). The membrane comprises a lipid bilayer, integral membrane proteins and a membrane skeleton (Fig. 1). Integral proteins (glycophorin and Band 3 proteins) are tightly bound to the membrane through hydrophobic interactions in the bilayer (Lux, 1979; Mohandas, 1991; Mohandas & Chasis, 1993). A filamentous network of proteins is anchored to the bilayer by the integral proteins. This network has three principal components: spectrin, actin, and protein 4.1 (Mohandas & Chasis, 1993). The membrane skeleton proteins interact with the lipid bilayer and transmembrane proteins to give the red cell membrane its strength and integrity (Tse & Lux, 1999). The peripheral membrane proteins are located on the cytoplasmic surface of the lipid bilayer and can be readily released from the membrane by simple manipulation of the ionic strength of the milieu or variation in the concentrations of other proteins (Mohandas & Chasis, 1993). Besides control of cell shape, the cytoskeletal proteins have also roles in organization of specialized membrane domains, and attachment to other cells and substrates (Cimen, 2008).

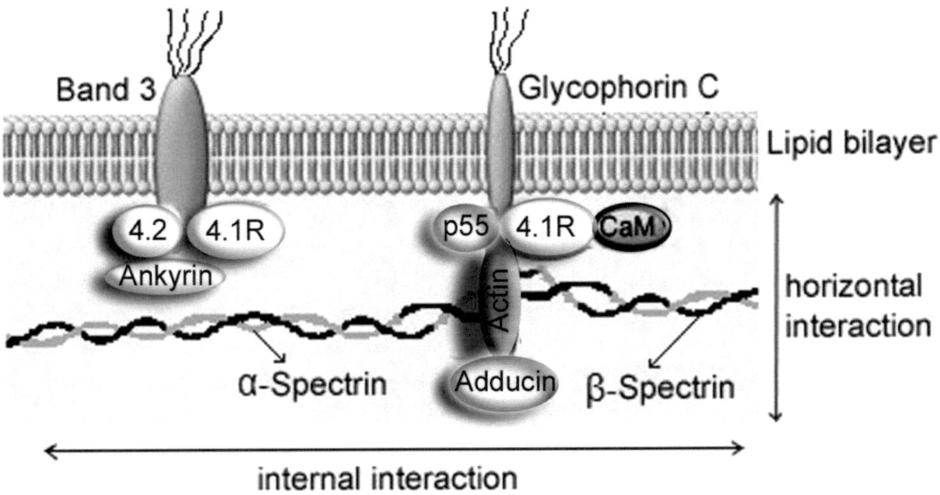

Fig. 1. The structure of erythrocyte membrane.

All lipids in the mature erythrocyte are found in the membrane bilayer and consist of phospholipid and cholesterol in 1.2:1 molar ratio. Approximately one-half of the fatty acids in the membrane are unsaturated (Telen & Kaufman, 1999). Interestingly, outer surface lipids exchange freely with the plasma lipid compartment (Bunn, 1991). In addition, the structure of the lipid bilayer is critical to the cytoskeletal network organization within the erythrocyte (Smith et al., 2005). Disruption of the interaction between components of the red cell membrane skeleton at any contact point may cause loss of structural and functional integrity of the membrane. There accepted to be two types of interactions: vertical interactions between the membrane skeleton and the lipid bilayer, and horizontal interactions among components that form the membrane skeleton meshwork. The important links in the vertical interaction involve band 3, ankyrin, spectrin and protein 4.2. The critical horizontal interactions occur between the α and β spectrins, β spectrin and protein 4.1, and protein 4.1 and actin (Morris & Lux, 1995).

Spectrin functions like a coiled spring able to stretch and snap back as the erythrocyte squeezes through capillaries, swells and shrinks, and is distorted by shear stresses. Spectrin attaches to the membrane via protein 4.1R and ankyrin. This confers sufficient tensile strength to withstand mechanical stresses and adequate flexibility to change shape as needed (Eber & Lux, 2004). The flexible, biconcave shape enables erythrocytes to squeeze through narrow capillaries. The erythrocytes need to endure both the micro and macrocirculatory environment. The rheological properties of erythrocytes microstructure play important roles in microcirculation, and also blood flow in large arteries. Microscopic mechanisms can be connected to the macroscopic behaviors of the blood and transferred by means of a blood viscosity model based on blood structure to the macroscopic behaviors of the blood (Yilmaz & Gundogdu, 2008).

Glucose, the only fuel utilized by erythrocytes, is primarily metabolized via anaerobic glycolysis. Following facilitated diffusion, glucose is immediately converted to glucose-6 phosphate. Approximately 80–90% percent is then converted to lactate via the glycolytic pathway. The remaining 10% undergoes oxidation via the pentose phosphate shunt. Glucose metabolism effectively maintains glutathione in the reduced form thereby protecting hemoglobin sulfhydryl groups and erythrocyte membranes from oxidation. A significant portion of the adenosine triphosphate (ATP) generated by glycolysis is spent in operating the sodium potassium pump necessary to reserve the cytoplasmic ionic milieu thus preventing colloidal osmotic lysis. In addition, some metabolic energy is expended on maintenance and repair of the red cell membrane (Bunn, 1991).

2. Erythrocytes, oxidative stress and aging

Mature, circulating erythrocytes have a finite life span. Each day, less than 1% of these cells are destroyed and replaced by virtually identical numbers of new cells. The molecular mechanism that determines removal of aged or damaged erythrocytes from the circulation remains unknown, but probably involves recognition of senescence antigens by phagocytes (Volpe, 1993). It has proposed that the major senescence antigen in aged erythrocytes is derived from the band 3 protein, the main transmembrane glycoprotein in erythrocytes. Other possible mechanisms for erythrocyte aging include mechanical fatigue, ATP depletion, calcium accumulation, and the generation of reactive oxygen species (ROS) (Feher et al., 2006). Erythrocytes experience continuous oxidative insult by being exposed to endogenous and exogenous ROS. ROS, which damage proteins and initiate lipid peroxidation, can be generated either inside erythrocytes through the hemoglobin oxidation pathway or outside. Although the erythrocyte contains an extensive antioxidant defense system, oxidative damage of membrane proteins and lipids contributes to the senescence of normal erythrocytes and results in a shorter life span for pathological cells.

The major source of intracellular ROS in the erythrocyte is autoxidation of oxyhemoglobin, which generates superoxide and produces hydrogen peroxide (H_2O_2). Catalase and glutathione peroxidase (GSHPx) scavenge most of the H_2O_2 generated in the cells. Degradation of the heme moiety takes place in conjunction with the reaction of H_2O_2 with hemoglobin. In addition, even small concentration of H_2O_2 generated during the autoxidation of oxyhemoglobin contributes to heme degradation. Heme degradation is, therefore, expected to take place in the erythrocyte when the antioxidant enzymes are not able to eliminate all the H_2O_2 (Snyder et al., 1985; Prokopiva et al., 2000; Feher et al., 2006).

One of the well established mechanisms of mechanical impairment of the erythrocyte is oxidative damage (Fig.2). Erythrocyte deformability is determined by cellular geometry, cytoplasmic viscosity of erythrocyte (hemoglobin concentration), and viscoelastic properties of the erythrocyte membrane. Membrane viscoelasticity is in turn determined by erythrocyte membrane skeleton, which is mainly a spectrin network attached to the integral proteins.

Oxidative reactions that start in the lipid components (i.e. lipid peroxidation) lead to the formation of cross-linkages within the membrane skeletal proteins or hemoglobin, increasing membrane viscosity. Additionally, oxidative damage may affect transport processes through the erythrocyte membrane, affecting the cell geometry and cytosolic viscosity (Feher et al., 2006; Aydogan et al., 2008).

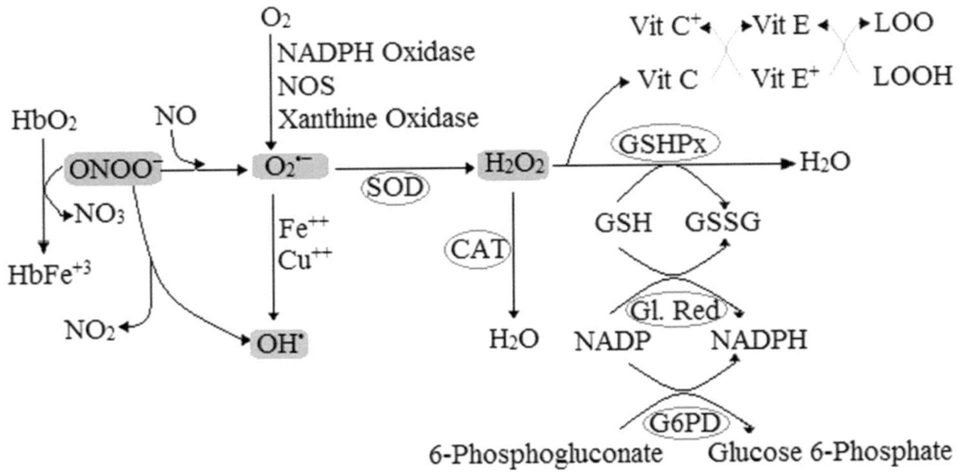

Fig. 2. Free radical metabolism in human erythrocytes.

The general consensus appears to be that the aging process is multifactorial and that ROS are a contributing factor. Particularly two phenomena are of particular concern: the deleterious effects of ROS and the formation of reactive carbonyl compounds related to the glycation reaction, involved in the acceleration of molecular and tissue aging processes. The ROS theory of erythrocyte aging has been widely accepted, yet it lacks direct supporting evidence, and the extent of ROS contribution remains uncertain.

The balance between ROS production and antioxidant defences determines the degree of oxidative stress. Unfortunately, the activity of these systems declines during aging, so the consequences of this stress include modification to to cellular components. Following the ROS mediated oxidation of sugar and membrane lipids through a complex and still unclear cascade of reactions. Carbonyl compounds are very reactive small molecules which can be considered a key oint in the propagation and amplification of the aging process. Carbonyl reactive compounds are able to form adducts commonly known as CO-proteins (proteins bearing carbonyl groups) with structural proteins lipoproteins, enzymes and with DNA, causing alterations in their biological activity thrugh a whole of chemical raction steps in all known as glycation reaction.

Glycation (or glycosylation) reaction is a reaction between reducing sugars, or other carbonyl group bearing molecules, and free amino groups of protein, leading to the formation of abnormal products, namely Advanced Glycation End Products (AGEs, cross-linked proteins). AGEs are very toxic for the cells, as they are very rich in double bonds which can interact irreversibly with biological substrates, leading to a loss of their physiological function. The result of cross-linking is a loss of physiological function, loss of genome information, and consequently senescence.

3. General effects of carnosine

L-Carnosine (B-alanyl-L-histidine) is a naturally occurring dipeptide and present in food. It is also commonly present in mammalian tissues. Carnosine is found naturally in the body. The highest concentrations are present in long-lived cells; particularly in skeletal muscles, followed by the heart, cerebellum and brain. No carnosine is detectable in plasma, liver kidney, and lung. It is formed by carnosine synthetase enzyme. It is kept in equilibrium by carnosinase enzyme. However its levels within the tissues decline with age.

Its proper function still remains unknown, although many properties have been proposed including physiological buffer (helps maintenance of the pH balance in the muscles in heavy exercise), wound healing agent, antioxidant (prevents the modification of biomacromolecules thereby keeping their native functionality under oxidative stress), free-radical and active sugar molecule scavenger (prevents glycation and carbonylation of proteins), heavy metal chelator (especially copper and zinc), immunomodulator and antitumor agent (e.g. suppresses of proinflammatory and carcinogenic cytokine IL-8), and anti-aging compound (Aruoma et al., 1989; Quinn et al., 1992; Gariballa & Sinclair, 2000).

Carnosine is a naturally occurring antioxidant that is also an anti-glycating agent. It has the ability to suppress Advanced Glycation End Products (AGEs) and formation of reactive oxygen species (ROS). In a remarkable series of experiments, scientists have shown that carnosine rejuvenates cells as they approach senescence (McFarland & Holliday, 1994, 1999). As shown by experiments on fibroblast cultures, carnosine retains youthful appearance and growth patterns. Fibroblasts that went through many rounds of division, known as late-passage cells, displayed a disorganized, irregular appearance before ceasing to divide. However fibroblasts cultured with carnosine lived longer, retaining youthful appearance and growth patterns. But, interestingly, when they transferred the fibroblasts back to a medium lacking carnosine, the signs of senescence quickly reappeared. The scientists switched late-passage fibroblasts back and forth several times between the culture media. They consistently observed that the carnosine culture medium restored the juvenile cell phenotype within days, whereas the standard culture medium brought back the senescent cell phenotype (McFarland & Holliday, 1994, 1999). Another group tested the effect of carnosine on life span and indicators of senescence in senescence-accelerated mice. Carnosine added to drinking water distinctly improved the appearance of the aged mice, whose coat fullness and color remained much closer to that of young animals The carnosine medium also increases life span, even for old cells. In the same study carnosine extended the life span of the treated mice by 20% on average, compared to the control mice. Carnosine did not alter the 15 month maximum life span of the senescence-accelerated mice strain, but it did significantly raise the number of mice surviving to old age (Boldyrev et al., 1999; Yuneva et al., 1999).

The current knowledge about the mechanisms involved in the aging process and the defense mechanisms are described in some experiments. Particularly, two phenomena are of particular concern: The deleterious effects of reactive oxygen species and the formation of reactive carbonyl compounds related to the glycation reaction, involved in the acceleration of molecular and tissue aging processes. The powerful and effective action of carnosine is performed against all the elements that triggered the aging process and against all the phenomena that contribute to its propagation and amplification (Hipkiss & Chana, 1998; Tamba & Torreggiani, 1999).

The anti-aging actions of L-carnosine may be summarized as follows (Fig.3): Carnosine stops the oxidative damage acting as an antioxidant agent, a ROS scavenger agent, metal ions chelating agent and by expressing superoxide dismutase (SOD)-like activity. It inhibits the glycation reaction, by quenching carbonyl compounds and AGEs. It also prevents the cross-linking of the macromolecules and promotes modification in enzyme-mediated protein degradation.

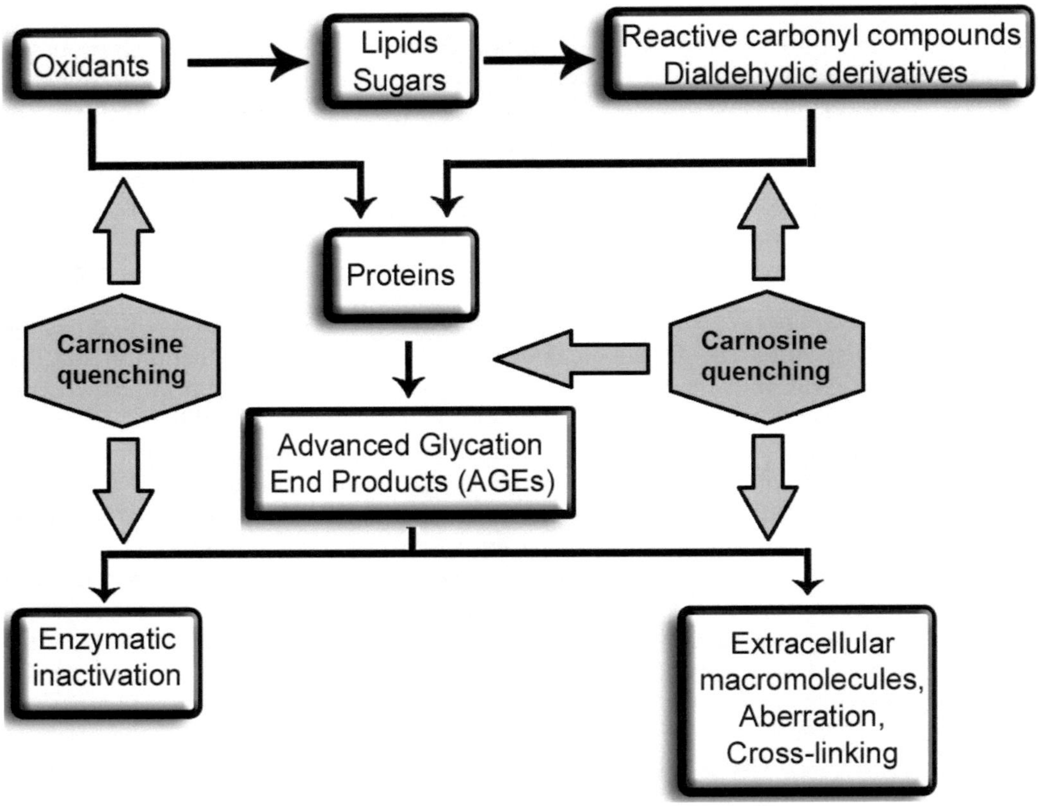

Fig. 3. The summary of sites of intervention of L-carnosine as anti-aging molecule.

Carnosine is widely believed to be an antioxidant which stabilizes and protects the cell membrane, and an oxygen free radical-scavenger (Kohen et al., 1988; Aruoma, Laughton et al., 1989; Boldyrev, Song et al., 1999). Specifically, as a water-soluble free radical scavenger it prevents lipid peroxidation within the cell membrane (Tamba & Torreggiani, 1999). It is thought to be a natural counterpart to lipid-soluble antioxidants such as vitamin E. Many antioxidants prevent free radicals from entering the tissues, but have no effect after this first line of defense is broken. Carnosine is not only effective in prevention, but it is also active after free radicals react to form other dangerous compounds. So, it protects the tissues from these damaging 'second-wave' chemicals. For example, it blocks a highly reactive lipid peroxidation end-product called malondialdehyde (MDA) (Kohen et al., 1988; Aruoma et al., 1989; Hipkiss et al., 1997; Hipkiss et al., 1998; Boldyrev, Song et al., 1999). MDA, if left uncontrolled, can cause damage to lipids, enzymes and DNA, and plays a part in the process of atherosclerosis, joint inflammation, cataract formation, and aging in general. Carnosine, by reacting and inactivating MDA, (Hipkiss et al., 1997) sacrifices itself in order to protect the amino acids on the protein molecule (Andrea et al., 2005). It has also the ability to reduce concentrations of thiobarbituric acid reactive substances (TBARS). Interacting with aldehydic lipid oxidation products, carnosine protects biological tissues from oxidation, since aldehydes can form adducts with DNA, proteins, enzymes, and lipoproteins, causing harmful alterations in their biological activity (Burcham et al., 2002). Many studies have demonstrated at tissue, cell and organel levels, that carnosine may prevent peroxidation of many model membrane system and also cell membrane, including erythrocytes (Boldyrev et al., 1997). Carnosine inhibits lipid oxidation by a combination of free radical scavenging and metal chelation. It has an ability to chelate prooxidative metals, such as copper, zinc and toxic heavy metals (lead, mercury, cadmium, nickel). Carnosine, as a dietary supplement, seems to have all the same chelating properties as EDTA (Hipkiss, 2005).

Carnosine can claim different properties performed at different steps of the whole aging process. Specifically, as a water-soluble free radical scavenger carnosine prevents lipid peroxidation within the cell membrane. Carnosine is not only effective in prevention, but it is also active after free radicals react to form other dangerous compounds. So, it protects the tissues from these damaging "second-wave" chemicals. It stops the oxidative damage acting as an antioxidant agent, a ROS scavenger agent, metal ions chelating agent and by expressing a superoxide dismutase (SOD) - like activity. It inhibits the glycation reaction, by quenching carbonyl compounds and AGEs. It prevents the cross-linking of the macromolecules (Hipkiss & Chana, 1998; Tamba & Torreggiani, 1999).

Age-related conditions that carnosine may be useful for: diabetes and its complications, neurological degeneration (Alzheimer´s, Parkinson´s, epilepsy, depression, schizophrenia, mild cognitive impairment, dementia and stroke), autistic spectrum disorders, cellular senescence in general cross-linking of the eye lens (cataracts), cross-linking of skin collagen (skin ageing), formation of AGEs, accumulation of damaged proteins, muscle atrophy, brain circulation deficit (stroke), and cardiovascular conditions (Boldyrev et al., 1997; Hipkiss, 2005).

One of the cardinal processes of aging, apart from the free-radical damage, is the process of glycosylation (or glycation). During normal metabolism, sugar aldehydes may react with the amino acids on the protein molecule, resulting in the formation of AGEs. AGEs are very toxic for the cells, which can react irreversibly with biological substrates leading to a loss of their physiological functions. Carnosine inactivates not only aldehydes and ketones, therefore reducing protein glycosylation and the formation of AGEs; but also already formed AGEs. Normally, AGEs are removed by scavenging macrophages which carry special receptors called RAGEs. Carnosine facilitates this process of elimination, by helping macrophages to better recognize the AGE molecules. Because of its anti-glycosylation actions, carnosine may be useful in treating or preventing diabetic complications such as cataract, neuropathy and kidney failure (Hipkiss & Chana, 1998).

With regard to oxidative modifications and erythrocyte demise, recent insights come from studies on their senescence suggesting that they can undergo a sort of apoptosis (Boas et al., 1998; Daugas et al., 2001). In particular, the apoptosis of erythrocytes was called eryptosis or erythroptosis depending on the injury pathway. The biological meaning and relevance of erythrocyte senescence and apoptosis, characterized by glycophorin A loss or phosphotidyl serine externalization respectively. However, although these are mainly referred to as critical events responsible for erythrocyte removal at the end of their life span, that subject is still a matter of debate (Daugas et al., 2001; Head et al., 2005; Pietraforte et al., 2007). For instance, the plethora of changes occurring in senescent and apoptotic erythrocytes under oxidative/nitrosative stress definitely comprises even biophysical changes, e.g. the loss of cell plasticity with impaired deformability associated with changes of cytoskeletal network assembly (Marchesi, 1985; An et al., 2002).

4. Effects of carnosine on erythrocyte rheology

The rheological properties of erythrocytes play important roles in microcirculation, and also blood flow in large arteries. Microscopic mechanisms can be connected to the macroscopic behaviors of the blood and transferred by means of a blood viscosity model based on blood structure to the macroscopic behaviors of the blood (Yilmaz & Gundogdu, 2008).

"Deformability" is the term generally used to characterize the erythrocyte's ability to undergo deformation during flow (Mohandas & Chasis, 1993). The deformation response of an erythrocyte to fluid forces is a complex phenomenon that depends on a number of different cell characteristics including membrane material properties (Lux, 1979), cell geometry, and cytoplasmic viscosity (Mohandas, 1991). Erythrocyte deformability is an important determinant of blood rheology, either in bulk flow conditions or microcirculation. Normal erythrocyte deformability is essential for proper tissue perfusion and oxygenation, as well as the normal survival of erythrocyte in the circulation.

Blood is a non-Newtonian fluid and its viscosity is therefore variable at any given temperature, depending on the shear rate. At low shear rate, erythrocytes can aggregate and form one-dimensional stacks-of-coins-like rouleaux or three-dimensional aggregates. This is because of the electrostatic repulsion of erythrocyte overcome by the present macromolecules which aggregate the cells. The process is reversible and particularly important in the microcirculation, since such rouleaux or aggregates can dramatically increase effective blood viscosity. Erythrocytes may also exhibit reduced deformability and stronger aggregation in many pathological situations, such as heart disease, hypertension, diabetes, malaria, and sickle cell anemia (Popel & Johnson, 2005).

The resistance of erythrocytes to hemolytic action is an integral parameter characterizing their integrity and viability as well as a criterion of their physiologically native state (Arzumanyan et al., 2008). Various factors can cause hemolysis of the erythrocytes, including a decreased ambient osmotic pressure, decreased pH, and oxidants (Ivanov, 1999; Pribush et al., 2002).

Oxidative damage in erythrocyte is one of the well established mechanisms of mechanical impairment. Erythrocytes are exposed to oxygen radicals continuously generated via the autoxidation of hemoglobin. In addition erythrocytes have relatively high levels of polyunsaturated fatty acids (PUFA), which are good substrates for peroxidation reactions. So due to the high iron content, relatively less antioxidant activities and high PUFA content the erythrocyte has a limited antioxidant defence.

Carnosine act as an antioxidant as well as a free-radical scavenger, which can protect and stabilize the cell membrane from non-enzymatic glycosylation and oxidation (Tamba & Torreggiani, 1999; Hipkiss & Brownson, 2000). In addition, carnosine also prevents protein glycation by using an enzyme that catalyses the splitting of interior peptide bonds in a protein (Quinn et al., 1992). Furthermore, the ability of carnosine to disintegrate the readily glycated protein was observed through the hydration and unfolding of deleterious reactions, such as the cross-linking of proteins (Seidler et al., 2004).

The significant role of L-carnosine in maintaining erythrocyte physiology under oxidative stress has been demonstrated previously by Aydogan et al (Aydogan et al., 2008). In that study blood from 3 and 10 months old rats had been used. L-carnosine improved erythrocyte deformability significantly in healthy erythrocytes independent of age. L-carnosine also significantly improved deformability in damaged erythrocytes as well both in the young and old rats (Fig.4). This study provided the first evidence for importance of carnosine in maintaining normal erythrocyte properties and to protect them from oxidative damage induced by H_20_2 administration under in vitro conditions. This observation was in favor of the idea that L-carnosine supplementation might be used to improve erythrocyte quality.

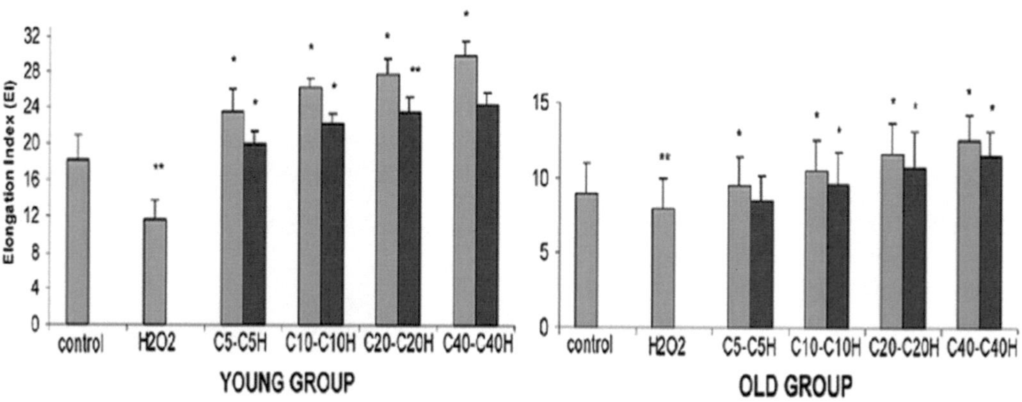

Fig. 4. Erythrocyte elongation indexes (EI) in control, treated with H_2O_2 and different concentrations of L-carnosine (5–40 mM) groups. Values are presented as mean ± SD, $n = 10$ for each group, * $p < 0.05$ when compared to H_2O_2, ** $p < 0.05$ when compared to control. "C" and "H" respectively indicates L-carnosine and H_2O_2 applications. The numbers following the letter "C" show carnosine concentrations. Reproduced from Aydogan et al. 2008 (Aydogan et al., 2008).

Another study from the same group showed that in vivo carnosine supplementation can be used to protect the erythrocytes from oxidative or peroxidative damage (Yerer et al., 2010). Sodium nitroprusside (SNP), which is a potent hypotensive agent, had been used to induce oxidative/nitrosative damage. Nitric oxide (NO) is a signaling molecule of major importance modulating not only the function of the vascular wall but also that of blood cells, such as platelets and leukocytes. The synthesis of NO in the circulation has been attributed mainly to the vascular endothelium. Erythrocytes have been demonstrated to carry a non-functional nitric oxide synthase (NOS) and due to their huge hemoglobin content have been assumed to metabolize large quantities of NO. However, more recently erythrocytes have been identified to reversibly bind, transport, and release NO within the cardiovascular system. This function of erythrocytes on NO metabolism also reflects the importance of oxidative damage via peroxinitrite. Oxidative and nitrosative damage to membrane erythrocyte membrane leads to the impairment of biorheological properties of the blood (Yerer et al., 2010). It is already known that NO increased either in pathological conditions and treatments with NO derivatives increase lipid peroxidation in the membrane of the erythrocytes (Yerer et al., 2004). When L-carnosine was given to rats intraperitoneally before the induction of oxidative damage by sodium nitroprusside, this prevented the increase in malondialdehyde (MDA), glutathione peroxidase (GSH-Px), and superoxide dismutase (SOD) (Fig.5A,B,C) activities. The changes in erythrocyte elongation indexes were in parallel as expected with these observations (Fig.5D). Carnosine application also significantly increased the erythrocyte elongation indexes that had already decreased by sodium nitroprusside (Yerer et al., 2004).

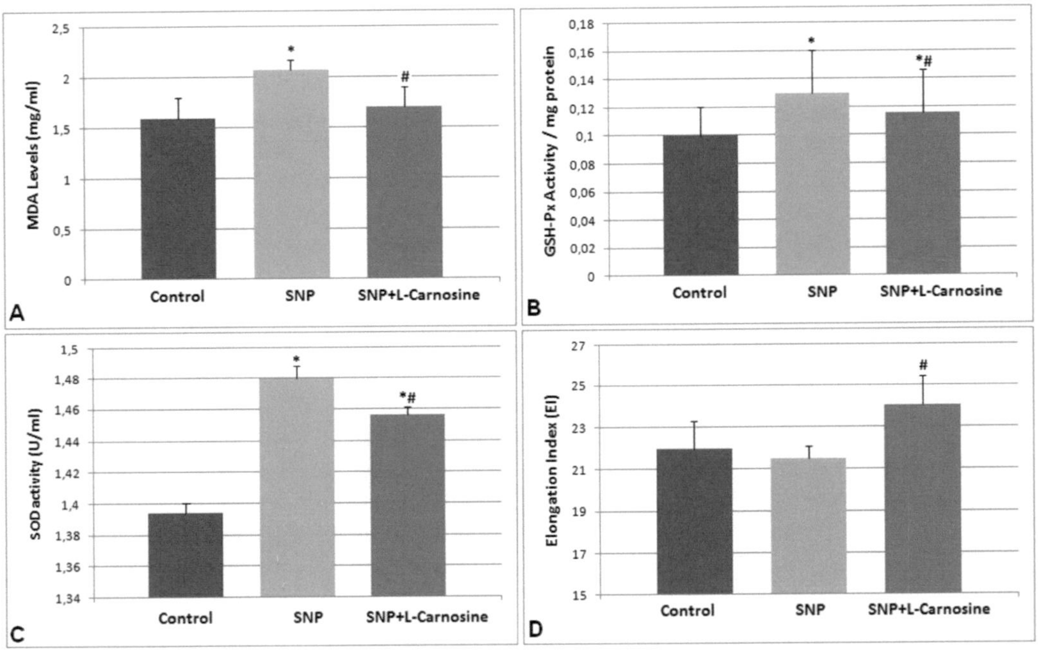

Fig. 5. A: Malondialdehyde (MDA) levels reflecting the lipid peroxidation. B: Glutathione peroxidase (GSH-Px) enzyme activity. C: Superoxide dismutase (SOD) enzyme activity. D: Elongation indexes (EI) reflecting erythrocyte deformability. *: significantly different from the control, #: significantly different from the sodium nitroprusside (SNP) group. Reproduced from Yerer et al 2010 (Yerer et al., 2010).

Similarly Arzumanyan et al have demonstrated that homocysteic acid (HCA) provokes oxidative stress in erythrocytes and decreases their hemolytic resistance, whereas the natural antioxidant carnosine protects erythrocytes from its toxic effect (Arzumanyan et al., 2008). Actually this should be taken into account when assessing the states of patients with chronic hyperhomocysteinemia. Homocysteine and the product of spontaneous homocysteine oxidation, namely HCA, are important risk factors for neurodegenerative and cardiovascular diseases (Jacobsen, 1998). The prooxidant effects of homocysteine and HCA on cell structures possibly occur via both the glutamate receptors (Vladychenskaya et al.,

2006) and the activation of NO synthase or inhibition of Na^+/K^+ ATPase (Arzumanyan et al., 2008). It is known that erythrocytes are capable of accumulating homocysteine and excreting it into the extracellular medium (Preibisch et al., 1993; Schlussel et al., 1995). Changes in the ambient osmotic pressure, pH, and oxidant levels are among the various factors causing hemolysis of erythrocytes. The resistance of erythrocytes to hemolytic action is an integral parameter characterizing their integrity and viability as well as a criterion of their physiologically native state. The investigators determined the level of free radicals in erythrocytes flow cytometrically and observed again that carnosine has a preventive effect on the harmful effects of HCA. The group tested any possible effects on erythrocytes by both osmotic and acid hemolysis (caused by hydrochloric acid) methods. The maximal number of cells hemolyzed osmotically by the end of the process remained the same. HCA increased the rate of acid erythrocyte hemolysis by 18–25%, whereas carnosine decreased the hemolysis rate to 80% of the control value irrespective of the presence or absence of HCA in the sample. The data from the study of Arzumanyan et al provided evidence for: (a) the preincubation of erythrocytes with homocysteic acid (HCA) considerably increases the hemolysis rate, (b) whereas carnosine prevents the hemolytic effect of HCA. The authors claim that the protective effect of carnosine had a pronounced dose-dependent manner.

Hemorheological properties are easily modified by glucose-induced oxidation and glycation. Carnosine prevents protein glycation by using an enzyme that catalyses the splitting of interior peptide bonds in a protein (Quinn et al., 1992). Furthermore, the ability of carnosine to disintegrate the readily glycated protein was observed through the hydration and unfolding of deleterious reactions, such as the cross-linking of proteins (Seidler et al., 2004). Another hemorheological in vitro study, conducted by Nam et al. on erythrocytes incubated in glucose-rich media, revealed the beneficial effects after addition of carnosine (Nam et al., 2009). In that study erythrocytes were incubated in glucose-rich media with different concentrations of carnosine. Also, defective erythrocytes due to hyperglycemia were incubated in autologous plasma with different concentrations of carnosine. When there was no carnosine in glucose-rich solution, both the erythrocyte deformability and aggregability significantly decreased. The degree of impairment in erythrocyte deformability and aggregability was proportional to the glucose-concentration. However, through the addition of carnosine to glucose solutions, the impairment of erythrocyte deformability and aggregability gradually diminished. To examine the rejuvenating function of carnosine, same researchers incubated erythrocytes, which were exposed to hyperglycemia-associated oxidative stress, in plasma that was supplemented with carnosine. As the carnosine concentration increased, the deformability of impaired erythrocytes slightly increased. Nam et al. also suggested that by increasing the incubation time, the deformability could be further increased. However, an increase in the carnosine concentration could cause echinocytic change in the shape of erythrocytes due to hyperosmolarity. During the same experiment researchers also investigated the aggregability of the erythrocytes. As the carnosine concentration increased in plasma, the aggregation index (AI) of impaired erythrocytes increased in a concentration-dependent manner. In addition, the increase in erythrocyte aggregability was also strongly dependent upon the incubation time, and the effect of carnosine was more prominent on aggregation than deformability. Thus, longer incubation periods for erythrocytes might increase erythrocyte aggregability up to the value of the control. The results of mentioned study reveal that the presence of carnosine effectively prevented rheological alterations due to glucose-induced oxidation and glycation in a concentration-dependent manner (Nam et al., 2009).

Diabetes mellitus is a disease characterized by insulin deficiency. It is known that oxidative stress plays an important role in physiopathology of chronic complications in diabetes. Since the structure of carnosine closely resembles that of the preferred glycation sites in proteins, the glycated sites may be occupied by carnosine, which, in turn, results in the rejuvenation of hemorheological characteristics. It is commonly known that most anti-oxidants prevent free radicals from binding the proteins but have no effect after protein binds with the free radicals. Yapıslar and Aydogan have investigated the effects of experimental diabetes on erythrocytes in rats (Yapislar & Aydogan, 2011). In that in vivo study erythrocyte deformability indexes and NO levels were decreased and MDA levels were found to be increased in diabetic group. Erythrocyte deformability abilities are reduced as a result of lipid peroxidation in erythrocyte membrane under diabetic condition (Yapislar & Aydogan, 2011; Nam et al., 2009). On the other hand, decrease in endothelium nitric oxide production might be responsible in endothelial dysfunction seen in diabetic vascular complications. NO is thought to cause oxidative and nitrosative damage to the erythrocyte. NO is a crucial component for erythrocytes which maintains different biological functions within the circulation. However, the excessive amounts of NO can trigger the oxidative and nitrosative damage especially to erythrocytes which leads to the impaired tissue perfusion (Yerer et al., 2010; Yapislar & Aydogan, 2011). Recent findings on the ability of carnosine to interact with guanylate cyclase heme also reflect the importance of this molecule in endogenous regulation of this enzyme over heme molecule (Severina et al., 2000). The data from the above mentioned study (Yapislar & Aydogan, 2011) revealed that carnosine application to diabetic rats significantly reversed the erythrocyte deformability and reduced the lipid peroxidation under diabetic conditions (Fig.6).

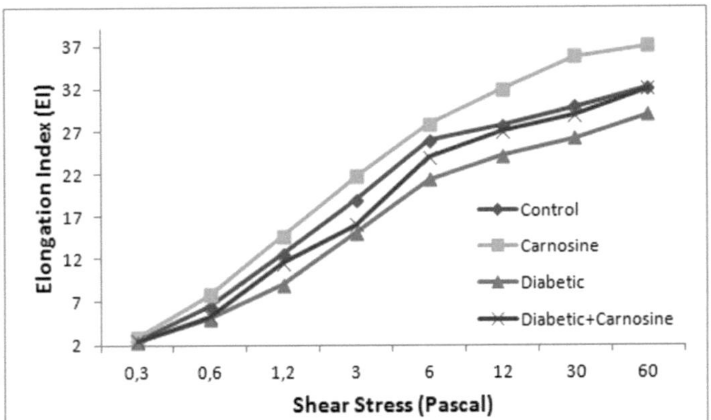

Fig. 6. Elongation indexes reflecting erythrocyte deformability after L-carnosine application in experimental diabetic rats at different shear stress rates. Reproduced from Yapislar and Aydogan 2011(Yapislar & Aydogan, 2011).

Aydogan et al. also recently studied deformability, aggregability, and osmotic fragility properties of healthy rat erythrocytes following incubation with L-carnosine (Aydogan et al., 2010) (article submitted). The data revealed that L-carnosine has a dose dependent positive effect on RBC deformability and aggregability. In the presence of carnosine, erythrocytes showed also an increased ability to resist hemolysis. This dipeptide appears to be rejuvenating or to improve erythrocyte quality and mechanical properties.

5. Conclusion

Carnosine is a natural and nontoxic compound. It has a high bio-availability and is lack of side effects. The beneficial properties of this dipeptide appear to be rejuvenating or to improve quality and mechanical properties of healthy erythrocytes. L-carnosine supplemention also can be used to protect them from several conditions or damages in survival of RBC in the circulation. Furthermore, use of carnosine after the pathology has occurred also helps to improve the deteriorated hemorheological status. These effects can be related to its antioxidant, free-radical scavenger, antiglycation and buffering properties.

L-carnosine helps healthy erythrocytes to fight agains oxidative stress and improve their survival in microcirculation. Supplementation with carnosine has rejuvenating effects on the healthy erythrocytes. It protects erythrocytes from oxidative stress occurring due to exposure to harmful conditions, including nitrosative stress, and glucose-induced oxidative stress and glycation. These beneficial effects of L-carnosine are dose and possibly incubation time dependent. Besides, damaged erythrocytes, as in the condition of experimental diabetes, also seem to improve following carnosine application. Carnosine performs an apparent rejuvenating function for hemorheologically damaged cells.

L-carnosine therefore seems to have crucial biological functions on erythrocytes which need to be identified with further investigations. In the light of the above mentioned studies in the literature it can be suggested that:

a. Carnosine can be used as for maintaining normal erythrocyte properties in healthy subjects and to improve the erythrocyte quality and survival.
b. L-carnosine can be used as a supplement in diabetes. It can recover microvascular circulation problems by increasing erythrocyte deformability, can reduce the risk of atherosclerosis and cardiovascular disease in diabetes by increasing NO levels, can protect cells and tissues against harmful effect of lipid peroxidation by decreasing lipid peroxidation and can be used as a multi-functional antioxidant in the treatment of diabetes mellitus to prevent the complications of diabetes.
c. There is a possibility of L-carnosine to be used for its protective effects on nitric oxide donor pharmaceutical damages in the circulation.
d. L-carnosine might be used as a pharmaceutical drug for treatment of malignant tumors, sepsis, asthma, migraine, i.e. pathologies which are associated with increasing the NO levels.
e. Moderate concentrations of carnosine might be further explored as potential therapeutic agents for pathologies that involve hemorheological modification.
f. Further experiments are in progress and it is expected that carnosine supplementation will become much more widespread during the next years.

6. References

An, X.; Lecomte, M.C.; Chasis, J.A.; Mohandas, N. & Gratzer, W. (2002). Shear-response of the spectrin dimer-tetramer equilibrium in the red blood cell membrane. *J Biol Chem,* Vol.277, No.35,pp.31796-31800.

Andrea, R.G.; Andrea, C.; Paolo, R. & Gianfranco, B. (2005). Carnosine and carnosine-related antioxidants: A review. . *Curr Med Chem.,* Vol.12, No.20,pp.2293-2315.

Aruoma, O.I.; Laughton, M.J. & Halliwell, B. (1989). Carnosine, homocarnosine and anserine: could they act as antioxidants in vivo? *Biochem J*, Vol.264, No.3,pp.863-869.

Arzumanyan, E.S.; Makhro, A.V.; Tyulina, O.V. & Boldyrev, A.A. (2008). Carnosine protects erythrocytes from the oxidative stress caused by homocysteic acid. *Dokl Biochem Biophys*, Vol.418,pp.44-46.

Aydogan, S.; Artis, A.S. & Basaran, E. (2010). A possible new role of L-carnosine as rejuvenating agent for improvement of erythrocyte quality and mechanical properties. 3rd Antiaging Congress. Ankara, Turkey June 2010, pp.17.

Aydogan, S.; Yapislar, H.; Artis, S. & Aydogan, B. (2008). Impaired erythrocytes deformability in H(2)O(2)-induced oxidative stress: protective effect of L-carnosine. *Clin Hemorheol Microcirc*, Vol.39, No.1-4,pp.93-98.

Benz, E.J., Jr. (2010). Learning about genomics and disease from the anucleate human red blood cell. *J Clin Invest*, Vol.120, No.12,pp.4204-4206.

Boas, F.E.; Forman, L. & Beutler, E. (1998). Phosphatidylserine exposure and red cell viability in red cell aging and in hemolytic anemia. *Proc Natl Acad Sci U S A*, Vol.95, No.6,pp.3077-3081.

Boldyrev, A.; Song, R.; Lawrence, D. & Carpenter, D.O. (1999). Carnosine protects against excitotoxic cell death independently of effects on reactive oxygen species. *Neuroscience*, Vol.94, No.2,pp.571-577.

Boldyrev, A.A.; Stvolinsky, S.L.; Tyulina, O.V.; Koshelev, V.B.; Hori, N. & Carpenter, D.O. (1997). Biochemical and physiological evidence that carnosine is an endogenous neuroprotector against free radicals. *Cell Mol Neurobiol*, Vol.17,No.2,pp.259-271.

Bunn, H.F. (1991). Pathophysiology of the anemias. *Harrison's Principle of Internal Medicine*,pp.1514-1518.

Burcham, P.C.; Kaminskas, L.M.; Fontaine, F.R.; Petersen, D.R. & Pyke, S.M. (2002). Aldehyde-sequestering drugs: tools for studying protein damage by lipid peroxidation products. *Toxicology*, Vol.181-182,pp.229-236.

Cimen, M.Y. (2008). Free radical metabolism in human erythrocytes. *Clin Chim Acta*, Vol.390,No.1-2,pp.1-11.

Daugas, E.; Cande, C. & Kroemer, G. (2001). Erythrocytes: death of a mummy. *Cell Death Differ*, Vol.8,No.12,pp.1131-1133.

Desouky, O.S. (2009). Rheological and electrical behavior of erythrocytes in patients with diabetes mellitus. *Romanian J. Biophys.* , Vol.19,No.4,pp.239-250.

Eber, S. & Lux, S.E. (2004). Hereditary spherocytosis--defects in proteins that connect the membrane skeleton to the lipid bilayer. *Semin Hematol*, Vol.41,No.2,pp.118-141.

Feher, G.; Koltai, K.; Kesmarky, G.; Szapary, L.; Juricskay, I. & Toth, K. (2006). Hemorheological parameters and aging. *Clin Hemorheol Microcirc*, Vol.35,No.1-2, pp.89-98.

Gariballa, S.E. & Sinclair, A.J. (2000). Carnosine: physiological properties and therapeutic potential. *Age Ageing*, Vol.29,No.3,pp.207-210.

Guyton, A.C. & Hall, J.E. (2000). Transport of oxygen and carbon dioxide in the blood and body fluids. In: *Textbook of medical physiology*,pp.463-473, W.B. Saunders. Philadelphia, PA.

Head, D.J.; Lee, Z.E.; Poole, J. & Avent, N.D. (2005). Expression of phosphatidylserine (PS) on wild-type and Gerbich variant erythrocytes following glycophorin-C (GPC) ligation. *Br J Haematol*, Vol.129,No.1,pp.130-137.

Hipkiss, A.R. (2005). Glycation, ageing and carnosine: are carnivorous diets beneficial? *Mech Ageing Dev*, Vol.126,No.10,pp.1034-1039.

Hipkiss, A.R. & Brownson, C. (2000). Review: A possible new role for the anti-ageing peptide carnosine. *Cell. Mol. Life Sci.,* Vol.57pp.747-753.

Hipkiss, A.R. & Chana, H. (1998). Carnosine protects proteins against methylglyoxal-mediated modifications. *Biochem Biophys Res Commun,* Vol.248,No.1,pp.28-32.

Hipkiss, A.R.; Preston, J.E.; Himswoth, D.T.; Worthington, V.C. & Abbot, N.J. (1997). Protective effects of carnosine against malondialdehyde-induced toxicity towards cultured rat brain endothelial cells. *Neurosci Lett,* Vol.238,No.3,pp.135-138.

Hipkiss, A.R.; Worthington, V.C.; Himsworth, D.T. & Herwig, W. (1998). Protective effects of carnosine against protein modification mediated by malondialdehyde and hypochlorite. *Biochim Biophys Acta,* Vol.1380,No.1,pp.46-54.

Ivanov, I.T. (1999). Low pH-induced hemolysis of erythrocytes is related to the entry of the acid into cytosole and oxidative stress on cellular membranes. *Biochim Biophys Acta,* Vol.1415,No.2,pp.349-360.

Jacobsen, D.W. (1998). Homocysteine and vitamins in cardiovascular disease. *Clin Chem,* Vol.44,No.8 Pt 2,pp.1833-1843.

Kohen, R.; Yamamoto, Y.; Cundy, K.C. & Ames, B.N. (1988). Antioxidant activity of carnosine, homocarnosine, and anserine present in muscle and brain. *Proc Natl Acad Sci U S A,* Vol.85,No.9,pp.3175-3179.

Lux, S.E. (1979). Dissecting the red cell membrane skeleton. *Nature,* 281, Vol.5731,No.pp.426-429.

Marchesi, V.T. (1985). Stabilizing infrastructure of cell membranes. *Annu Rev Cell Biol,* Vol.1,No.pp.531-561.

McFarland, G.A. & Holliday, R. (1994). Retardation of the senescence of cultured human diploid fibroblasts by carnosine. *Exp Cell Res,* Vol.212,No.2,pp.167-175.

McFarland, G.A. & Holliday, R. (1999). Further evidence for the rejuvenating effects of the dipeptide L-carnosine on cultured human diploid fibroblasts. *Exp Gerontol,* Vol.34,No.1,pp.35-45.

Mohandas, N. (1991). The red blood cell membrane.In: *Hematology: Basis, Principles and Practice.* R. Hoffman, E. J. Benz, S. J. Shattil, B. Furie & H. J. Cohen,pp.264-269, Churchill-Livingstone.New York.

Mohandas, N. & Chasis, J.A. (1993). Red blood cell deformability, membrane material properties and shape: regulation by transmembrane, skeletal and cytosolic proteins and lipids. *Semin Hematol,* Vol.30,No.3,pp.171-192.

Morris, M.B. & Lux, S.E. (1995). Characterization of the binary interaction between human erythrocyte protein 4.1 and actin. *Eur J Biochem,* Vol.231,No.3,pp.644-650.

Nam, J.H.; Kim, C.B. & Shin, S. (2009). The effect of L-carnosine on the rheological characteristics of erythrocytes incubated in glucose media. *Korea-Australia Rheology Journal,* Vol.21,No.2,pp.103-108.

Nohl, H. & Stolze, K. (1998). The effects of xenobiotics on erythrocytes. *Gen Pharmacol,* Vol.31,No.3,pp.343-347.

Pietraforte, D.; Matarrese, P.; Straface, E.; Gambardella, L.; Metere, A.; Scorza, G.; Leto, T.L.; Malorni, W. & Minetti, M. (2007). Two different pathways are involved in peroxynitrite-induced senescence and apoptosis of human erythrocytes. *Free Radic Biol Med,* Vol.42,No.2,pp.202-214.

Popel, A.S. & Johnson, P.C. (2005). Microcirculation and Hemorheology. *Annu Rev Fluid Mech,* Vol.37,No.,pp.43-69.

Preibisch, G.; Kuffner, C. & Elstner, E.F. (1993). Biochemical model reactions on the prooxidative activity of homocysteine. *Z Naturforsch C,* Vol.48,No.1-2,pp.58-62.

Pribush, A.; Meyerstein, D. & Meyerstein, N. (2002). Kinetics of erythrocyte swelling and membrane hole formation in hypotonic media. *Biochim Biophys Acta,* Vol.1558,No.2,pp.119-132.

Prokopiva, V.D.; Bohan, N.A.; Johnson, P.; Abe, H. & Boldyrev, A.A. (2000). Effect of carnosine and related compounds on the stability and morphology of erythrocytes from alcoholics. *Alcohol and Alcoholism,* Vol.35,No.1,pp.44-48.

Quinn, P.J.; Boldyrev, A.A. & Formazuyk, V.E. (1992). Carnosine: its properties, functions and potential therapeutic applications. *Mol Aspects Med,* Vol.13,No.5,pp.379-444.

Schlussel, E.; Preibisch, G.; Putter, S. & Elstner, E.F. (1995). Homocysteine-induced oxidative damage: mechanisms and possible roles in neurodegenerative and atherogenic processes. *Z Naturforsch C,* Vol.50,No.9-10,pp.699-707.

Seidler, N.W.; Yeargans, G.S. & Morgan, T.G. (2004). Carnosine disaggregates glycated alpha-crystallin: an in vitro study. *Arch Biochem Biophys,* Vol.427,No.,1,pp.110-115.

Severina, I.S.; Bussygina, O.G. & Pyatakova, N.V. (2000). Carnosine as a regulator of soluble guanylate cyclase. *Biochemistry (Mosc),* Vol.65,No.7,pp.783-788.

Smith, C.; Marks, A.D. & Lieberman, M. (2005). *Mark's Basic Medical Biochemistry* (edition).Lippincott Williams & Wilkins, Philadelphia.

Snyder, L.M.; Fortier, N.L.; Trainor, J.; Jacobs, J.; Leb, L.; Lubin, B.; Chiu, D.; Shohet, S. & Mohandas, N. (1985). Effect of hydrogen peroxide exposure on normal human erythrocyte deformability, morphology, surface characteristics, and spectrin-hemoglobin cross-linking. *J Clin Invest,* Vol.76,No.5,pp.1971-1977.

Tamba, M. & Torreggiani, A. (1999). Hydroxyl radical scavenging by carnosine and Cu(II)-carnosine complexes: a pulse-radiolysis and spectroscopic study. *Int J Radiat Biol,* Vol.75,No.9,pp.1177-1188.

Telen, M.J. & Kaufman, R.E. (1999). The mature erythrocyte.In. J. P. Greer & J. Foerster,pp.217-247, Lippincott Williams & Wilkins.Philadelphia.

Tse, W.T. & Lux, S.E. (1999). Red blood cell membrane disorders. *Br J Haematol,* Vol.104,No.1,pp.2-13.

Vladychenskaya, E.A.; Tyulina, O.V. & Boldyrev, A.A. (2006). Effect of homocysteine and homocysteic acid on glutamate receptors on rat lymphocytes. *Bull Exp Biol Med,* Vol.142,No.,1,pp.47-50.

Volpe, E.P. (1993). Blood and circulation.In: *Biology and Human Concerns.* W. C. Dubuque,pp.253–265, William C Brown Pub

Yapislar, H. & Aydogan, S. (2011 Vol.85,No.). Effect of carnosine on erythrocyte deformability in streptocotocin induced diabetic rats; relationship between carnosine and nitric oxide. ESCHM Congress. Munich, Germany, June 2011, pp:144.

Yerer, M.B.; Aydogan, B. & Aydogan, S. (2010). Sodium nitroprusside-induced oxidative damage on erythrocytes: Protective role of carnosine. *Series on Biomechanics,* Vol.25,No. 1-2,pp.194-198.

Yerer, M.B.; Yapislar, H.; Aydogan, S.; Yalcin, O. & Baskurt, O. (2004). Lipid peroxidation and deformability of red blood cells in experimental sepsis in rats: The protective effects of melatonin. *Clin Hemorheol Microcirc,* Vol.30,No.2,pp.77-82.

Yilmaz, F. & Gundogdu, M. (2008). A critical review on blood flow in large arteries; relevance to blood rheology, viscosity models, and physiologic conditions. *Korea-Australia Rheology J.,* Vol.20,pp.197-211.

Yuneva, M.O.; Bulygina, E.R.; Galant, S.C.; Kramarenko, G.G.; Stvolinsky, S.L.; Semyonova, M.L. & Boldyrev, A.A. (1999). Effect of carnosine on age-induced changes in senescence accelerated mice. *Journal of Anti-Aging Medicine,* Vol.2,No.4,pp.337-342.

7

Soluble Guanylate Cyclase Modulators in Heart Failure

Veselin Mitrovic* and Stefan Lehinant
Kerckhoff-Klinik gGmbH, Bad Nauheim, Germany

1. Introduction

Despite significant advances in the modern diagnosis and pharmacologic and nonpharmacologic therapy for heart failure, with a reduction of mortality of more than 50%, long-term prognosis of the disease still is poor and, often, with uncertain outcome [1, 2].

The great expectations set in vasopeptidase inhibitors, tumor necrosis factor–α antagonists, metalloproteinase inhibitors, endothelin antagonists, and adenosine A1-receptor antagonists could not be verified by findings as has been shown in large-scale clinical trials. The calcium sensitizer levosimendan, the vasopressin V2-receptor antagonist tolvaptan, and the natriuretic peptide (NP) nesiritide only partially fulfilled the expectations. There remains an urgent unmet need for new therapies with new drugs and new modes of action.

Drugs that modulate soluble guanylate cyclase (sGC) and cyclic guanosine 3′, 5′-monophosphate (cGMP) levels are emerging as promising therapies for heart failure. The sGC activator cinaciguat and sGC stimulators riociguat and BAY 60-4552 as modulators of sGC are promising drugs with favorable effects such as vasodilatation; inodilation; and antiproliferative, antiapoptotic, and antiremodeling effects through protein kinase G-type and phosphodiesterases as well as calcium ion channels [3].

Cinaciguat (BAY 58-2667) is a novel molecule that activates regulatory sites on both the α and β subunits of sGC, a key signal transduction enzyme that synthesizes cGMP in response to binding of nitric oxide. Cinaciguat has a unique feature, to activate sGC independently of NO and of the prosthetic heme group. Cinaciguat is even more potent if the heme group is oxidized and insensitive to NO.

Riociguat (BAY 63-2521) is a direct stimulator of sGC in vitro and in vivo that is independent from NO, the endogenous activator of the enzyme. Moreover, in the presence of NO, it enhances the effect of NO [4, 5••]. In previous clinical studies, riociguat revealed beneficial effects and good tolerability in patients with pulmonary hypertension [6] and patients with severe heart failure [7].

This article summarizes the pathophysiologic relevance and therapeutic potential of the sGC–cGMP signalling system in acute and chronic heart failure.

* Corresponding Author

2. Guanylate cyclase pathway

Cyclic guanosine 3′, 5′-monophosphate is a second messenger that plays a role in various crucial physiologic pathways, including cardiovascular homeostasis, cellular growth and contractility, inflammation, sensory transduction, and neuronal plasticity and learning [8]. Guanylate cyclases (GC) are enzymes that catalyze the conversion of guanosine-5'-triphosphate to cGMP. The GC-family includes both membrane-bound and soluble isoforms that are expressed in nearly all cell types. Membrane-bound particulate guanylate cyclase (pGC) serves as a receptor for NPs, whereas plasmatic sGC acts as a receptor for biological messenger NO. Subsequently, cGMP effectors include cGMP-dependent protein kinases, cGMP-regulated phosphodiesterases, and cyclic nucleotide-gated ion channels (Fig. 1) [9].

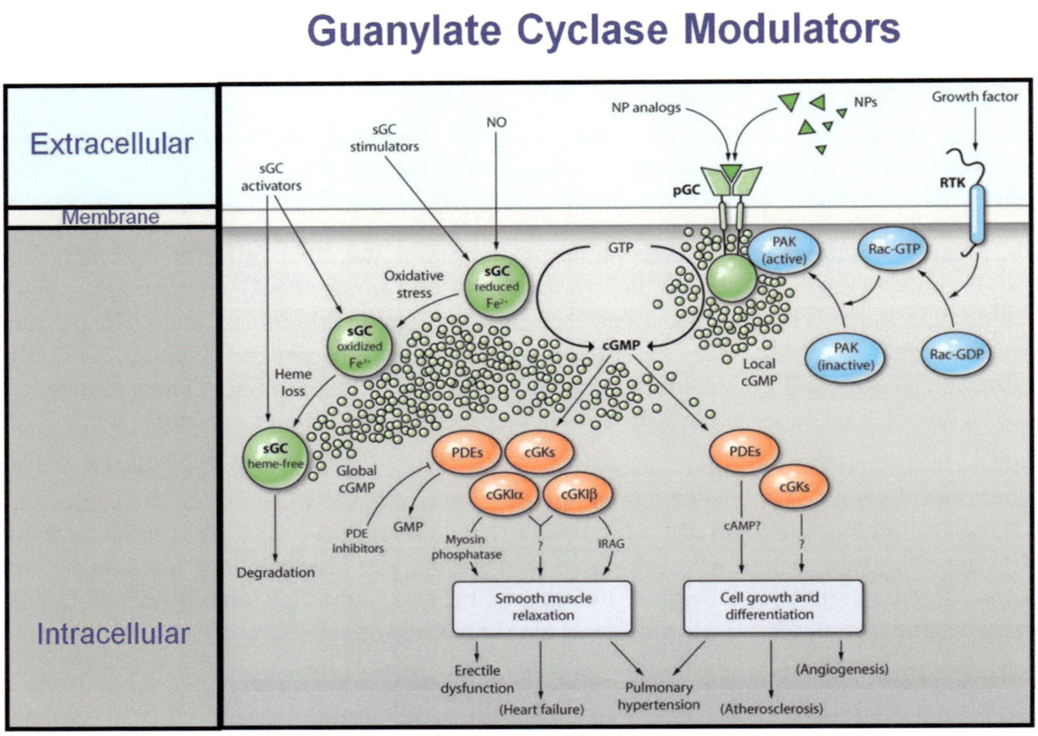

Barbara Kemp-Harper, Sci. Signal., 2008

NO – nitric oxide; NP – natriuretic peptide; RTK; pGC – particulate guanylate cylase; sGC – soluble guanylate cyclase; cGMP – cyclic guanosine 3′, 5′-monophosphate; PDEs – phosphodiesterases; cGKs – cGMP-dependent protein kinases; GTP – guanosine-5'-triphosphate; PAK; GDP; IRAG – inositol 1,4,5-trisphosphate receptor I-associated protein; cAMP – cyclic adenosine monophosphate.

Fig. 1. sGC- and pGC-cGMP signalling pathways. cGMP acts through cGMP effectors including cGMP-dependent protein kinases, cGMP-modulated cation channels, and cGMP-regulated phosphodiesterases that hydrolyze cyclic nucleotides.

Both the NO-sGC-cGMP pathway and the NP-pGC-cGMP pathway are disordered in a range of cardiovascular conditions, including acute decompensated heart failure (ADHF) [10••].

The NP–pGC signalling pathway has been shown to play an important role as a compensatory mechanism that reduces neurohumoral activation in heart failure. pGC contains an extracellular ligand-binding domain and an intracellular catalytic domain connected by a single transmembrane domain [11]. At least seven pGC family members have been identified and sequenced (GC-A to GC-G).

In humans, NPs constitute a family of at least four identified members: atrial natriuretic peptide (ANP) and B-type natriuretic peptide (BNP), of myocardial origin; C-type natriuretic peptide (CNP), derived from the endothelial cells; and urodilatin, produced in the kidneys [12, 13]. The GC-A binding ligands ANP and BNP are produced predominantly in the cardiac atria and ventricles and released in the circulation in response to hypervolemia, as seen, for example, in congestive heart failure, to regulate blood pressure and body fluid homeostasis. An activation of a GC-A binding domain by ANP and BNP results in cGMP increase mediating hypotensive and cardioprotective actions through increased natriuresis, inhibition of the renin-aldosterone pathway, as well as vasorelaxant, antifibrotic, antihypertrophic, and lusitropic effects [10••, 13].

In patients with heart failure, the described compensatory response to NPs is disturbed due to markedly altered distribution and degradation of the NPs [14]. It has been demonstrated that there is an inadequate neurohumoral response to volume/sodium overload not only in advanced stages of heart failure, but also in patients with only very mild symptoms of the disease [15].

As for the NO–sGC–cGMP pathway, in conditions of oxidative stress that typically occur with cardiovascular diseases, the NO production is reduced. On the other hand, the NO degradation and neutralization by oxidants such as superoxide is excessively increased, contributing to an overall NO deficiency [3, 16•]. Additionally, the oxidation of the heme group on sGC impairs the enzyme bioavailability and responsiveness to endogenous NO and exogenous nitrovasodilators reducing the activation of this signalling pathway even further [3].

The described disruption of physiologic signalling response in patients with heart failure builds the rationale for new therapeutic agents that target these GC pathways.

Several novel drugs that induce the pGC–cCMP pathway include NP analogues nesiritide and ularitide. Both compounds show natriuretic, diuretic, and vasodilating effects [17, 18]. While there is good evidence of positive short-term hemodynamic effects of nesiritide in ADHF [19], there still is controversy regarding its safety risks, including renal dysfunction and long-term mortality [20], that needs to be addressed in future trials. Ularitide currently is being evaluated and is showing promising effects on preserving renal function in patients with decompensated heart failure. These results also need to be further investigated in lager trials [21, 22].

Although the activation of sGC and pGC cascades produce the same second messenger, it has been demonstrated that the effects of cGMP differ in dependence of the origin of production. The probable explanation for this effect are different locations of GCs within the cardiac myocytes with sGC being mainly located in the cytosol and pGC being mainly found in subsarcolemmal areas [23]. This concept of compartmentalization of cGMP is particularly interesting for predicting effects of novel therapies modulating either one or the other signaling pathway. Thus, the effects of synthetic NP analogues like nesiritide or ularitide as ligands of pGC differ slightly from therapeutic agents that target sGC like cinaciguat.

In the following section, we focus on the cGC–cGMP pathway and its activation through a novel NO-independent activator cinaciguat (BAY 58-2667).

3. sGC signalling pathway

NO is a key signaling molecule in a variety of physiologic processes in mammals. NO is produced endogenously from the amino acid L-arginine by the enzyme NOS. There are different NOS isoforms that were isolated from the brain, vascular endothelium, and macrophages [24]. Endothelial NOS (eNOS) is a Ca^{2+}- and calmodulin-dependent NO-synthase that originally was identified as constitutive in vascular endothelial cells. Activation of eNOS is induced by two basic pathways: sheering forces produced by blood flow and endothelial receptors for a variety of ligands like bradykinin, acetylcholine, adenosine, and other vasoactive substances. Both pathways cause a release of calcium with subsequent eNOS activation. eNOS produces nitric oxide and activates sGC located in the adjacent vascular smooth muscle cells, thereby increasing levels of cGMP and inducing vasorelaxation. This mechanism is thought to play a major role in the regulation of vascular tone and blood pressure [24].

Reduced bioavailability and/or responsiveness to endogenous NO contribute to the development of cardiovascular diseases [3, 10••]. Organic nitrates, such as nitroglycerin, and other NO-donor drugs, known as vasodilators, as they showed beneficial effects on a variety of cardiovascular diseases including various anginal syndromes and congestive heart failure. During short-term therapy, nitrates rapidly improve hemodynamics by increasing levels of cGMP in the vascular smooth muscle cell with resultant peripheral arteriolar and venous vasodilatation providing a decrease in filling pressures and systemic vascular resistance, and thereby lowering myocardial oxygen consumption [25]. However, one of the major limitations of nitrates is the development of dose-related tolerance in long-term treatment, as well as nonspecific interactions of NO with other biological molecules [3, 26]. Furthermore, despite potent short-term symptoms relief, there is no clear evidence of long-term mortality reduction in patients with cardiovascular disease [3].

To understand the difference between the mechanisms of actions of traditional therapeutics like nitrates and new compound like cinaciguat, it is important to outline the structure of their receptor sGC. sGC is a heterodimer consisting of an α- and a heme-containing β-subunit. NO only can induce sGC upon binding to its reduced Fe^{2+} heme moiety. It its oxidized state, sGC heme strongly reduces its affinity for the sGC heme binding site, often resulting in a subsequent loss of the prosthetic heme group. Its loss renders the enzyme insensitive to endogenous and exogenous NO [3, 27, 28].

Cardiovascular diseases like atherosclerosis, diabetes, and hypertension are associated with a high degree of oxidative stress. During oxidative stress, reactive oxygen species (ROS) interfere with NO–sGC signalling pathway by reducing NO bioavailability and by oxidizing the sGC heme moiety, thereby leading to sGC degradation.

Unlike conventional nitrovasodilators, two novel therapeutic groups can induce sGC in its NO-insensitive state, so-called sGC-activators and sGC-stimulators. sGC-activators like cinaciguat induce the soluble guanylate cyclase in its NO-insensitive, oxidized ferric (Fe^{3+}) heme-free state. On the other hand, sCG-stimulators like YC-1, BAY 41-2272, CFM-1571, A-350619, and riociguat enhance the affinity of sGC to already very low levels of NO, thereby producing synergistic effects with NO (Fig. 2).

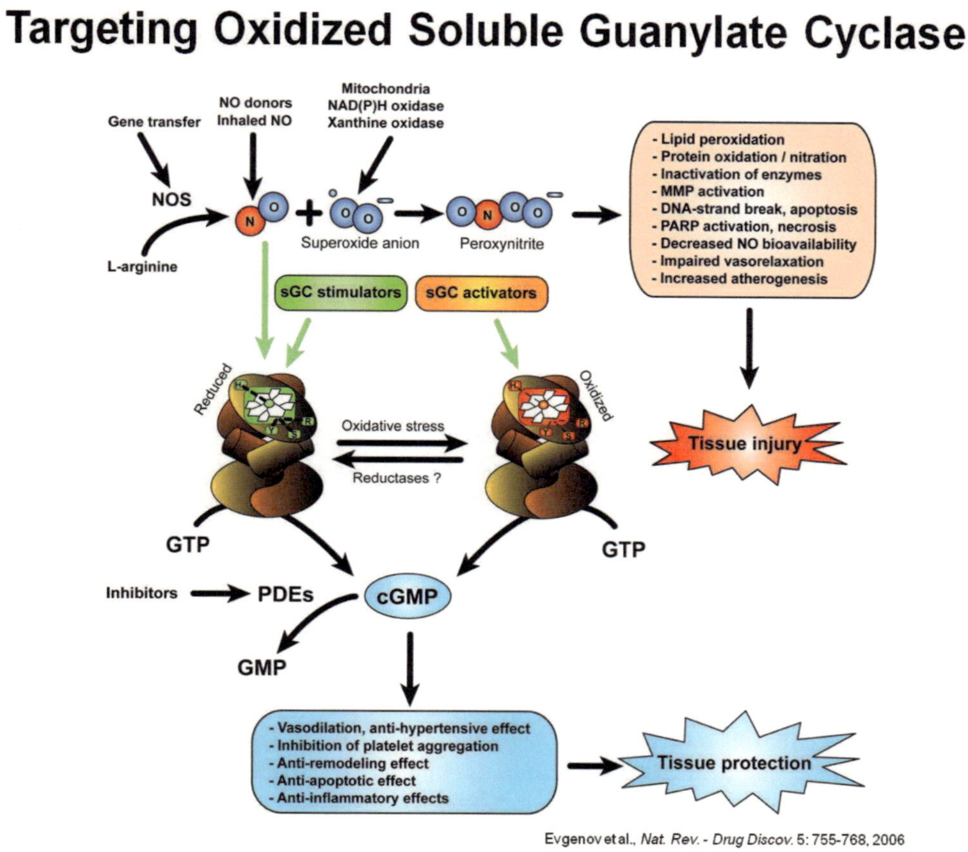

NO—nitric oxide; GTP—guanosine-5'-triphosphate; sGC—soluble guanylate cyclase; PDEs—phosphodiesterases; GMP—guanosine monophosphate; MMP; PARP; NOS—nitric oxide synthase.

Fig. 2. NO-sGC-cGMP signalling pathway. Mechanism of action of sGC stimulators and sGC activators. See text for explanation.

4. Cinaciguat: Clinical benefits in decompensated heart failure

Cinaciguat, the first of a new class of sGC activator, is in early clinical development for the treatment of acute decompensated heart failure (ADHF). The few preclinical and clinical data show that it has great potential as an effective substance for treatment of ADHF. In animal experimental studies, the cardiorenal effects of intravenous cinaciguat 0.1 or 0.3 μg/kg/min were evaluated [29•, 30]. Cinaciguat potently unloads the heart by reducing arterial pressure, pulmonary arterial pressure, and pulmonary capillary wedge pressure (PCWP), thereby increasing the cardiac output (CO), renal blood flow, and glomerular filtration rate.

Initial studies in healthy volunteers have demonstrated the clinical utility of cinaciguat. A favorable safety profile and efficacy were documented in lower doses of 50 to 250 μg/h for up to 4 hours [31••].

After initial dose finding, cinaciguat was evaluated in a nonrandomized, uncontrolled, proof-of-concept study that included 33 patients with ADHF of functional classes NYHA III and IV and PCWP of 18 mm Hg or greater using a starting dose of 100 μg/h, which could be uptitrated to final doses of 50 to 400 ng/h depending on hemodynamic response.

Patients were categorized as responders to the new substance if the PCWP decreased by 4 mm Hg or more compared with baseline. The responder rate was 53% after 2 hours, 83% after 4 hours, and 90% after 6 hours. The proportion of patients reporting improvements in dyspnea scores increased during and after 6 hours of cinaciguat intravenous infusion [32, 34••].

Initial results showed promising evidence of the therapeutic potential and safety of cinaciguat: continuous intravenous administration was well tolerated and increased the potent venous and arterial dilation, which led to significant cardiac preload and afterload reduction and increased cardiac index. Compared with baseline, a 6-hour infusion of cinaciguat led to significant reductions in mean pulmonary artery pressure (-6.5 mm Hg), PCWP (7–8 mm Hg), mean right arterial pressure (-2.9 mm Hg), PVR (-43.4 dynes/s/cm^{-5}), and SVR (-597 dynes/s/cm^{-5}), while increasing heart rate by 4.4 bpm and CO by 1.68 L/min [33, 34••].

Of 60 patients, 13 reported 14 drug-related treatment-emergent adverse events of mild to moderate intensity, most commonly hypotension.

In a placebo-controlled, randomized, double-blind, multicenter, international phase 2b study, the safety and efficacy of intravenous cinaciguat as an add-on to standard therapy was investigated in 159 patients with ADHF. Hemodynamic effects were monitored via Swan-Ganz thermodilution catheter (Edwards Lifesciences, Irvine, CA) in patients with NYHA functional class III and IV HF and PCWP of 18 mm Hg or greater [35].

Cinaciguat dose was titrated from 100 to a maximum of 600 μg/h for the first 8 hours and was then maintained for up to 40 hours. Primary end point was a change in PCWP after 8 hours compared with placebo; secondary end points included hemodynamic and safety parameters, organ protection, and 30-day mortality.

In this study, 159 patients on stable standard therapy were enrolled within 48 hours after hospital admission to receive placebo or cinaciguat. The new substance caused a rapid and sustained decrease in the primary end point PCWP, increased CO, and decreased pulmonary vascular resistance (PVR) without changing heart rate. No adverse effects on cardial or renal function or 30-day mortality were observed despite increased occurrence of several cases of oligosymptomatic hypotension at high doses of cinaciguat, which led to prematurely termination of the study [35].

Under low dosage of intravenous Cinaciguat, a phase 2b study (COMPOSE EARLY) currently is recruiting participants to investigate the efficacy and tolerability of Cinaciguat (150 μg/h, 100 μg/h, 50 μg/h) [35]. The results are expected within the next 2 years.

5. Riociguat: Clinical utility in heart failure and pulmonary hypertension

Riociguat has shown its unique mechanism of action through simultaneous lowering systemic vascular resistance (SVR) and PVR in a phase 2 trial in patients with pulmonary arterial hypertension (PAH) and chronic thromboembolic pulmonary hypertension (CTEPH) [6].

The trials confirmed the expected pharmacologic mode of action, which is consistent with the properties of a sGC stimulator and showed significant effects on pulmonary hemodynamics (decrease of PVR, increase of CO), echocardiographic parameters, N-terminal proBNP levels, and functional capacity (improvement in 6-minute walking distance) without major safety concerns. Improvements also were observed in NYHA functional class and Borg dyspnea score. Riociguat was well tolerated and had a favorable safety profile [6, 31••].

Based on these data, two randomized, placebo-controlled, phase 3 studies have begun: the CHEST-1 study (A Study to Evaluate Efficacy and Safety of Oral BAY63-2521 in Patients With CTEPH) in patients with CTEPH and the PATENT-1 trial (A Study to Evaluate Efficacy and Safety of Oral BAY63-2521 in Patients With Pulmonary Arterial Hypertension) for patients with PAH. Both studies will be followed by open long-term studies (CHEST-2 and PATENT-2). Recruitment for CHEST-1 and PATENT-1 is ongoing. Results from the study program are expected in 2011.

Similar reduction of SVR and PVR was seen in a single-dose study in 42 patients with biventricular heart failure (LVEF $\leq$ 45%, pulmonary artery pressure mean $\geq$ 25 mm Hg, and PCWP $\geq$ 18 mm Hg) to evaluate the acute hemodynamic response to BAY 60-4552, a main metabolite of riociguat. Oral administration of doses from 1 to 10 mg was well tolerated and mediated a potent vasodilation. Biventricular preload and afterload were improved, subsequently resulting in a significant increase of cardiac index. Riociguat shows great promise for treatment in pulmonary hypertension associated with left ventricular systolic dysfunction on top of standard congestive heart failure therapy.

Currently, riociguat is being investigated in a multicenter study in patients with congestive heart failure and pulmonary hypertension (LEPHT study [A Study to Test the Effects of Riociguat in Patients With Pulmonary Hypertension Associated With Left Ventricular Systolic Dysfunction]).

6. Conclusions

Cyclic guanosine-3′,5′ monophosphate is a second messenger that plays a role in various physiologic signalling pathways. It is produced either by membrane-bound pGC or sGC. pGC is induced by NPs; sGC by NO. In cardiovascular diseases like ADHF, the physiological NO–sGC and NP–pGC signalling pathways are disrupted.

Cinaciguat, a novel NO-independent sGC activator, offers many advantages over traditional organic nitrates and other NO-donor drugs, whose use often is limited due to tolerance development, limited biometabolism, nonspecific interactions, lack of sGC activation in the absence of the sGC heme moiety, and lack of benefit in long-term mortality.

Cinaciguat is a novel sGC activator that binds to the NO-sensitive oxidized ferric (Fe^{3+}) or heme-free sGC, thus stimulating cGMP synthesis. In this way, the substance is effective under oxidative stress, which is present in many cardiovascular diseases.

Despite limited clinical data for cinaciguat, preliminary studies in patients with ADHF demonstrate a significant hemodynamic benefit and reduction of symptoms. Further studies are required to evaluate cinaciguat, in particular, because of its novel and promising mode of action. There is a need for studies that address long-term symptoms and mortality in a larger number of patients with ADHF.

Riociguat (BAY 63-2521) has been investigated in 14 clinical pharmacological studies confirming the mechanism of action of the compound as an sGC stimulator.

A proof-of-concept study in patients with pulmonary hypertension showed that sGC stimulation exerted by a single dose of riociguat had the expected favorable hemodynamic effects on subjects with pulmonary hypertension.

In a phase 2 study, riociguat, at doses between 1 mg three times daily and 2.5 mg three times daily, was administered for 12 weeks to 72 subjects with pulmonary arterial hypertension and chronic thromboembolic pulmonary hypertension.

Riociguat was generally safe and well tolerated and exerted significant and favorable effects on pulmonary hemodynamics and functional capacity. This was supported by evidence from echocardiography biomarker and functional class assessment.

7. Disclosures

No potential conflicts of interest relevant to this article were reported.

8. References

Papers of particular interest, published recently, have been highlighted as:
• Of importance
• • Of major importance

[1] Stuart S, MacIntyre K, Hole DJ, et al.: More 'malignant' than cancer? Five-year survival following a first admission for heart failure. Eur J Heart Fail 2001; 3(3): 315-322)

[2] Grigioni F, Potena L, Galiè N, et al.: Prognostic implications of serial assessments of pulmonary hypertension in severe chronic heart failure. J Heart Lung Transplant. 2006; 25: 1241-1246.

[3] Evgenov OV, Pacher P, Schmidt PM, et al.: NO-independent stimulators and activators of soluble guanylate cyclase: discovery and therapeutic potential. Nat.Rev.Drug Discov.2006.Sep.;5(9.):755.-68. 2006, 5:755-768

[4] Schermuly RT, Stasch JP, Pullamsetti SS, et al.: Expression and function of soluble guanylate cyclase in pulmonary arterial hypertension. Eur Respir J. 2008; 32: 881-891.

[5] • • Stasch JP, Hobbs AJ: NO-independent, haem-dependent soluble guanylate cyclase stimulators. Handb Exp Pharmacol. 2009; (191): 277-308.
This is an excellent overview of background of effects of NO-independent sGC stimulators.

[6] Ghofrani HA, Hoeper MM, Hoeffken G, et al.: Riociguat Dose Titration in Patients with Chronic Thromboembolic Pulmonary Hypertension (CTEPH) or Pulmonary Arterial Hypertension (PAH). Conference abstract. 2009 American Thoracic Society International Conference, San Diego, USA, 16-20 May 2009.

[7] Mitrovic V, Swidnicki B, Ghofrani A, et al.: Acute hemodynamic response to single oral doses of BAY 60-4552, a soluble guanylate cyclase stimulator, in patients with biventricular heart failure. Conference abstract. 4th International Conference on cGMP, Regensburg, Germany, 19-21 Jun 2009.
[8] Feil R, Kemp-Harper B: cGMP signalling: from bench to bedside. Conference on cGMP generators, effectors and therapeutic implications. EMBO Rep.2006.Feb.;7.(2):149.-53. 2006, 7:149-153
[9] Lucas KA, Pitari GM, Kazerounian S, et al.: Guanylyl cyclases and signaling by cyclic GMP. Pharmacol.Rev.2000.Sep.;52.(3):375.-414. 2000, 52:375-414
[10] •• Mitrovic V, Hernandez AF, Meyer M, et al.: Role of guanylate cyclase modulators in decompensated heart failure. Heart Fail.Rev.2009.Dec.;14(4):309.-19. 2009, 14:309-319. This is a first-time overview of effects of pGC and sGC modulators in patients with heart failure. Natriuretic peptides (nesiritide and ularitide) lead to an increase of cGMP through stimulation of pGC; however. sGC stimulators and activators lead to an increase of intracellular cGMP through modulation of soluble guanylate cyclase.
[11] Joseph L, Jr. Izzo, American Council on High Blood Pressure, and Henry R.Black: Hypertension Primer: The Essentials of High Blood Pressure 2003:Chapter A3, 8-13
[12] Burnett JC Jr.: Novel therapeutic directions for the natriuretic peptides in cardiovascular diseases: what's on the horizon. J.Cardiol.2006.Nov.;48.(5):235.-41. 2006, 48:235-241
[13] Lee CY, Burnett, JC Jr.: Natriuretic peptides and therapeutic applications. Heart Fail.Rev.2007.Jun.;12.(2):131.-42. 2007, 12:131-142
[14] Clerico A, Iervasi G, Pilo A.: Turnover studies on cardiac natriuretic peptides: methodological, pathophysiological and therapeutical considerations. Curr.Drug Metab.2000.Jul.;1(1):85.-105. 2000, 1:85-105
[15] Volpe M, Tritto C, De Luca N, et al.: Failure of atrial natriuretic factor to increase with saline load in patients with dilated cardiomyopathy and mild heart failure. J.Clin.Invest. 1991, 88:1481-1489
[16] • Pacher P, Beckman JS, Liaudet L: Nitric oxide and peroxynitrite in health and disease. Physiol Rev.2007.Jan.;87.(1):315.-424. 2007, 87:315-424
This paper describes the role of oxidative stress in cardiovascular disease.
[17] Atlas SA, Maack T: Effects of atrial natriuretic factor on the kidney and the renin-angiotensin-aldosterone system. Endocrinol.Metab Clin.North Am. 1987, 16:107-143
[18] van der Zander K, Houben AJ, Hofstra L, et al.: Hemodynamic and renal effects of low-dose brain natriuretic peptide infusion in humans: a randomized, placebo-controlled crossover study. Am.J.Physiol Heart Circ.Physiol.2003.Sep.;285.(3): H1206.-12.Epub.2003.May.8. 2003, 285:H1206-H1212
[19] Mills RM, LeJemtel TH, Horton DP, et al.: Sustained hemodynamic effects of an infusion of nesiritide (human b-type natriuretic peptide) in heart failure: a randomized, double-blind, placebo-controlled clinical trial. Natrecor Study Group. J.Am.Coll.Cardiol. 1999, 34:155-162
[20] Sackner-Bernstein JD, Skopicki HA, Aaronson KD: Risk of worsening renal function with nesiritide in patients with acutely decompensated heart failure. Circulation.2005.Mar.29.;111.(12.):1487.-91.Epub.2005.Mar.21. 2005, 111:1487-1491
[21] Luss H, Mitrovic V, Seferovic PM, Simeunovic D, et al. Renal effects of ularitide in patients with decompensated heart failure. Am.Heart J.2008.Jun.;155.(6.):1012.e1.-8. 2008, 155:1012-1018

[22] Mitrovic V, Seferovic PM, Simeunovic D, et al.: Haemodynamic and clinical effects of ularitide in decompensated heart failure. Eur.Heart J.2006.Dec.;27.(23):2823.-32.Epub.2006.Oct.30. 2006, 27:2823-2832

[23] Su J, Scholz PM, Weiss HR: Differential effects of cGMP produced by soluble and particulate guanylyl cyclase on mouse ventricular myocytes. Exp.Biol.Med.(Maywood.).2005.Apr;230.(4):242.-50. 2005, 230:242-250

[24] Knowles RG, and Moncada S: Nitric oxide synthases in mammals. Biochem.J. 1994, 298 (Pt 2):249-258

[25] Torfgard KE, Ahlner J: Mechanisms of action of nitrates. Cardiovasc.Drugs Ther. 1994, 8:701-717

[26] Packer M, Lee WH, Kessler PD, et al.: Prevention and reversal of nitrate tolerance in patients with congestive heart failure. N.Engl.J.Med. 1987, 317:799-804

[27] Foerster J, Harteneck C, Malkewitz J, et al.: A functional heme-binding site of soluble guanylyl cyclase requires intact N-termini of alpha 1 and beta 1 subunits. Eur.J.Biochem. 1996, 240:380-386

[28] Ignarro LJ, Adams JB, Horwitz PM, et al.: Activation of soluble guanylate cyclase by NO-hemoproteins involves NO-heme exchange. Comparison of heme-containing and heme-deficient enzyme forms. J.Biol.Chem. 1986, 261:4997-5002

[29] •Boerrigter G, Costello-Boerrigter LC, Cataliotti A, et al.: Targeting heme-oxidized soluble guanylate cyclase in experimental heart failure. Hypertension 2007. 49:1128–1133
The authors show that sGC activators act by an oxidized form of sGC, in contrast to sGC stimulators, which exert their effect through a reduced variant of sGC.

[30] Boerrigter G, Costello-Boerrigter LC, Cataliotti A, et al.: Targeting heme-oxidized soluble guanylate cyclase with BAY 58-2667 in experimental heart failure. BMC Pharmacology 2007. 7:P9

[31] •• Frey R, Muck W, Unger S, et al.: Pharmacokinetics, pharmacodynamics, tolerability, and safety of the soluble guanylate cyclase activator cinaciguat (BAY 58-2667) in healthy male volunteers. J Clin Pharmacol 2008.48:1400-1410
This is a first-time description of efficacy and safety of the sGC activator cinaciguat in healthy male volunteers.

[32] Lapp H, Mitrovic V, Franz N, et al.: BAY 58–2667, a soluble guanylate cyclase activator, improves cardiopulmonary haemodynamics in acute decompensated heart failure and has a favourable safety profile. BMC Pharmacology. 2007: 7:S9

[33] Mitrovic V, Lapp H, Franz N, et al.: The soluble guanylate cyclase activator cinaciguat (BAY 58-2667) has a favourable safety profile and improves cardiopulmonary haemodynamics in acute decompensated heart failure. Poster presented at Heart Failure 2008, 14–17 June, Milan, Italy.

[34] ••Lapp H, Mitrovic V, Franz N, et al.: Cinaciguat (BAY 58 2667) improves cardiopulmonary hemodynamics in patients with acute decompensated heart failure. Circulation. Published online May 18, 2009
This is a first-time description of the hemodynamic effects of the sGC activator cinaciguat in patients with decompensated heart failure as a new promising model for therapy.

[35] Erdmann E, Semigran MJ, Nieminen MS, et al.: Cinaciguat, a soluble Guanylate Cyclase Activator, unloads the heart in acute decompensated heart failure. Cinaciguat phase IIb abstract for ACC 2010.

8

Advantages of Catheter-Based Adenoviral Delivery of Genes to the Heart for Studies of Cardiac Disease

J. Michael O'Donnell
Program in Integrative Cardiac Metabolism, Center for Cardiovascular Research, and Department of Physiology and Biophysics, University of Illinois at Chicago, College of Medicine
USA

1. Introduction

With the advent and rapid advancement of genetically engineered methodologies (ie., cDNA, siRNA and transgenics), there has been an unprecedented acceleration in the identification of the underlying maladaptive processes of heart disease. New pharmaceutical and gene therapy strategies targeted at correcting these maladaptions show unprecedented promise. In particular, the transfer of exogenous cDNA or siRNA by viral based vehicles show great promise for both the overexpression or suppression, respectively, of the proteins linked to these maladaptations in heart. Indeed, the translation of these current viral based studies from animal models of cardiac disease to humans are now in clinical trials (Jessup et al., 2011; Hajjar et al., 2008; Jaski et al., 2009; Gwathmey et al., 2011). However, progress is slowed by weak and inefficient techniques for the transport and delivery of exogenous genes to the heart in animal and human.

Much like the transport of consumer goods across the country, the transport of exogenous genes to the heart requires both an efficient route of transport and an efficient delivery vehicle. This chapter briefly compares the efficiency of the various delivery routes to the heart, and we compare two of the more popular vehicles (adenovirus vs adeno-associated virus). We will argue that the adenoviral (Adv) delivery of genes by a catheter-based route provides considerable advantages for molecular based studies of heart disease. Alternatively, the emerging and less invasive adeno-associated vector (AAV) is better suited for therapeutic gene transfer in human. Several groups have demonstrated that simple systemic injection of the AAV-cDNA in rodents enables significant gene transfer and long-term expression of the targeted proteins in heart (see review Wasala et al., 2011). However, in larger animals and humans, the promise of this less invasive approach has not translated well. In larger mammals, gene transfer to the heart still requires an invasive catheter-based surgical procedure (White et al., 2011, Kaye et al., 2007; Hayase et al., 2005). Here, we will discuss some of these gene transfer strategies and their limitations.

We will also describe our surgical advancement to the conventional catheter-based technique for gene delivery to the heart. This approach significantly improves gene transfer to the heart and eliminates both virus accumulation and gene transfer to non-target organs in rat (O'Donnell et al., 2004, 2005, 2008, 2009). The earlier conventional form of this open-chest catheter-based approach has been used extensively to deliver the cDNA for the Ca^{2+}-ATPase, SERCA2a, to heart as a potential therapeutic strategy for the treatment of heart failure (Del Monte et al., 2002). While there are a number of reports that this strategy improves cardiac hemodynamics, function, and survival (Miyamoto et al., 2000; Del Monte et al., 2001), the results via our modified approach challenge this data and the safety of the treatment proposed for humans (O'Donnell et al., 2008). Our finding has recently been supported by a second report in transgenic mice overexpressing SERCA2a subjected to ascending aortic constriction (Pinz et al., 2011). Here, we briefly review this opposing data, and discuss conditions for this discrepancy, which require consideration as a safe and effective treatment strategy continues to evolve for clinical applications. The controversy of this therapeutic strategy, as it relates to the stage and model of the disease, is also discussed in a recent commentary by Sipido and Bangheluwe (Sipido et al., 2010).

2. Methods of gene delivery to the heart

The development of efficient techniques for direct in vivo gene transfer is important not only to support basic science studies in animal models, but also for gene therapy of heart disease in human. However, progress to date has been limited by difficulties in the available gene delivery systems (Prasad et al., 2011). Ideally, the gene delivery approach would be minimally invasive and provide a robust and homogenous transfection to the whole heart without an autoimmune or toxic side effect. To this end, several delivery approaches have been developed and examined both in animals and humans as illustrated in Figure 1. These methods include direct injection of the viral vehicle into (a) the pericardial sac, (b) the intramyocardial tissue, (c) the intraventricular chamber, (d) intravenous delivery, or (e) catheter-based delivery of the virus into the aortic root which enables delivery of the virus to the whole heart via the coronary arteries.

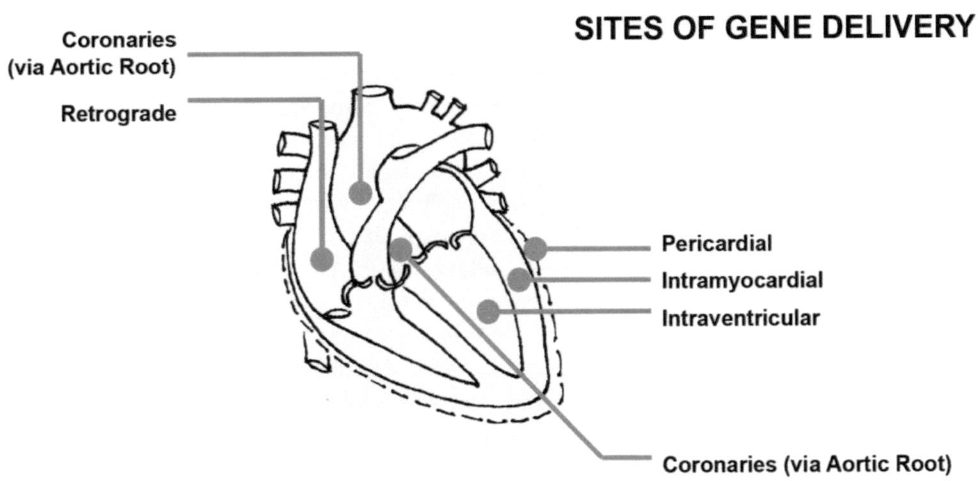

Fig. 1. Sites of gene delivery to the heart via viral_cDNA based methodologies. The highest level of gene transfer has been achieved by coronary perfusion of the heart via catheter-based delivery routes.

2.1 Routes of gene delivery

The different routes of viral delivery demonstrate different efficiencies of gene transfer and durations of gene expression in heart (Wasala et al., 2011). The direct injection of the viral-cDNA package into the heart tissue results in a very localized gene transfer at the site of injection (Svensson et al., 1999; Su et al., 2000). When an adenoviral vector is used, the expression peaks at one week and subsequently declines (Guzman et al., 1993). Similarly, intravenous injection of the adenoviral-cDNA package results in peak expression in heart within a week in adult rat and mice (Stratford-Perricaudet et al., 1992). However, unlike the localized injection, the intravenous injection results in widespread infection of peripheral tissue (liver, skeletal muscle, lung). Adenoviral gene transfer also results in an inflammatory response in the heart after 4-5 days, and the expression of the targeted protein is gone after a few weeks (Kass-Eisler et al., 1993). Therefore, studies must be completed within 3 days of gene transfer when the overexpression is maximal and the inflammatory response is minimal.

Unlike the adult mouse or rat model, intraventricular injection of the adenoviral-cDNA package into neonatal mouse hearts leads to the overexpression of exogenous gene for several months (2-12 mths) with no inflammatory response (Stratford-Perricaudet et al., 1992). This chronic overexpression is due to incorporation of the transferred gene into the animal's genome. However, the two month expression window in mice is often not long enough to study chronic models of heart disease, and infection of non-target tissue is still observed (Stratford-Perricaudet et al., 1992).

As an alternate method to intravascular or intraventricular administration, when the adenoviral-cDNA package is injected into the pericardial sac of adult rats, gene transfer is exclusively restricted to the pericardial cell layers (Fromes et al., 1999). However, injecting a mixture of collagenase and hyaluronidase together with the virus, leads to a somewhat larger diffusion (40%) of the transgene through the myocardial wall. The collateral effects of the collagenase / hyaluronidase are unclear.

The transfer of exogenous genes to the whole heart, in vivo, by the catheter-based approach has consistently demonstrated the most promising strategy. The approach was first described by Barr in 1994 (Barr et al., 1994). A catheter was inserted into the right carotid artery and advanced to the coronary ostia before injecting 1 ml of Adv.cmv.lacZ into the coronary artery. A cross section of heart stain for lacZ expression showed myocytes expressing the exogenous gene. However, infection was sparse and efficiency was <1%. An important advancement to the approach was presented by Hajjar's laboratory in 1998 (Hajjar et al., 1998). The viral solution was injected into the aortic root after first cross-clamping the aorta and pulmonary artery. This enabled both a high injection pressure and longer incubation periods prior to releasing the cross-clamp. Subsequent refinements to this basic approach have since yielded efficiencies as high as 40-80% in hamster (Ikeda et al., 2002), mouse (Champion et al., 2003; Iwatate et al., 2003), and rat (Ding et al., 2004). However, the approach still results in (a) infection of non-target tissue (liver, skeletal muscle, lung), (b) an inflammatory response within a week, and (c) some groups report that the level of gene transfer to the heart by the conventional approach is low (Wright et al., 2001; Ding et al., 2004; O'Donnell et al., 2005).

Nevertheless, several groups have demonstrated that the adenoviral delivery of exogenous genes to the heart by the catheter-based approach can enhance cardiac function and provide a potential therapeutic strategy for the treatment of heart disease. For a detailed discussion of the various trans-genes examined over the past decade, see the recent review by Wasala (Wasala et al., 2011). In brief, Hajjar's group has demonstrated in both rat and sheep models of heart failure that the overexpresson of SERCA2a leads to enhanced cardiac function, extended life span, and reduced arrhythmias (Miyamoto et al., 2000; Byrne et al., 2008). Similarily, the catheter-based delivery of an adenovirus carrying the phospholamban gene resulted in a significant change in left ventricular function (Hajjar et al., 1998). Ross has also demonstrated that coronary delivery of adenovirus carrying the cDNA for δ-sarcoglycan, in a sarcoglycan deficient hamster model of dilated cardiomyopathy, results in enhance left ventricular function (Ideda et al., 2002). Using a modified catheter-based technique, Maurice has shown that the overexpression of a β-adrenergic receptor significantly enhanced heart contractility and hemodynamic performance in rabbits (Maurice et al., 1999).

Cumulatively, these studies demonstrate the therapeutic utility of the catheter-based adenoviral delivery approach for the modulation of heart function, but a common limitation for these studies was that the overexpression of the exogenous gene was low in the heart, the transfer of the exogenous gene to peripheral organs was also observed, and cardiac inflammation was observed by one week. Furthermore, while the results proved promising, it is not completely resolved whether the functional improvement with the treatment strategy was a direct result of the targeted transgene or due to potential peripheral mechanisms.

Our group has since advanced the conventional catheter-based approach to reduced peripheral effects. This advanced approach results in highly efficient and global gene transfer to the whole heart with minimal infection of peripheral tissue. We've since used this catheter-based delivery approach to determine if the overexpression of the Ca2+-ATPase, SERCA1a, can be used as a therapeutic strategy for the treatment of cardiac hypertrophy and ischemia reperfusion. In support of other reports (Chen et al., 2004; Taluker et al., 2007), we found the strategy significantly improved post-ischemic recovery of cardiac function and metabolism in rat (O'Donnell et al., 2009). However, the strategy compromised cardiac function in the hypertrophic heart (O'Donnell et al., 2008). This finding contradicts the earlier reports which used the conventional catheter-based cross-clamp approach to delivery the cDNA for SERCA2a (Miyamoto et al., 2000; Del Monte et al., 2001; Byrne et al., 2008). Whether this discrepancy is related to (a) the higher level of gene transfer achieved by our approach (ie., a dose response), (b) the elimination of gene transfer to peripheral tissue by our approach, (c) the specific isoform of SERCA gene transferred (SERCA1 vs SERCA2), or (d) the stage of the disease model (early vs late stage heart failure) is unclear and discussed under section 4.5.

2.2 Vehicles of gene delivery

Equal to the selection of the delivery route is the selection of the viral vehicle used to deliver the exogenous cDNA. Several viral vectors are currently being investigated for gene delivery to provide either transient or permanent transgene expression. These include adenovirus (Adv), adeno-associated virus (AAV), retrovirus, lentivirus, and herpes simplex virus-1 (HSV-1). The Adv can carry a ~30 kb genome, and the expression of the exogenous gene is initially very high, reaching its maximal effect within the first 2-5 days, as discussed. While the adenovirus can efficiently transduce the myocardium, the vector is limited by short-term gene expression (2 weeks) and there is an immune response to viral proteins after five days (Gilgenkrantz et al., 1995) which can cause significant myocardial inflammation. Therefore, Adv is useful when a high level of expression is required, and studies can be completed before the inflammatory response.

The recombinant adeno-associated viral vectors (AAV) offers an attractive alternative. See the recent review by Reyes-Juarez and Zarain-Herzberg for a detailed discussion (Reyes-Juarez et al., 2011). In brief, the AAV (25 nm) is smaller than the conventional Adv adenovirus which enables the virus to cross the endothelial barrier with greater ease in rat and mouse (Xie et al., 2002; Dhu et al., 2003). Consequently, several groups have shown that simple intravenous or intramuscular injections yield highly efficient gene transfer to the heart or skeletal muscle (Zhu et al., 2005; Blankinship et al., 2004; Kawamoto et al., 2005). This makes delivery both minimally invasive and highly efficient, two important criteria toward controlling gene transfer. In addition, the AAV serotype is not pathogenic, there is little evidence of inflammation with use, and expression is long term (years) (Gregorevic et al., 2004; Aikawa et al., 2002). Unfortunately, as with the conventional adenovirus (Adv), expression of genes delivered via the AAV within non-target cells remains problematic causing deleterious side effects (Aikawa et al., 2002; Su et al., 2004). However, this cross-infection can be reduced by using specific serotypes of the AAV (AAV-1, 2, 5, 6, 7, 8, and 9). These serotypes have an array of tissue tropisms and binding characteristics (Zhu et al., 2005; Du et al., 2004) making the discovery of a cardiac specific AAV a promising strategy.

In rodent models, AAV has been delivered via the catheter-based coronary perfusion approach, direct myocardial injection, and intravenous delivery (Wasala et al., 2011). Svensson and colleagues delivered AAV-2_LacZ to adult mouse heart by coronary perfusion and direct injection (Svensson et al., 1999). While the expression of exogenous genes were minimal at 2 weeks, expression was robust at 8 weeks with 50% of the cardiomyocytes transduced by the trans-coronary perfusion. Similarily, Hoshijima reported the expression of genes persisted for 30 weeks in hamsters with AAV-2 (Hoshijima et al., 2002). Using a far less invasive approach, Gregorevic injected AAV-6 into the tail vein of adult mice and found extensive gene transfer to heart and skeletal muscles (Gregorevic et al., 2004). Xiao and colleagues reported similar high gene transfer to heart and skeletal muscle with intraperitoneal and/or intravascular injection of AAV-2 (Wang et al., 2005). Others have also shown that AAV-9 is 10 fold stronger than AAV-2 and 8 in transducing mouse heart (Bish et al., 2008; Inagaki et al., 2006), though this serotype also displays a strong tropism for gene transfer to off target organs including liver. However, in dividing/regenerative cells such as in liver, the expression of exogenous genes via AAV persist for only 1-2 months, while in non-dividing cells such as in heart, the expression is long-term.

To reduce the expression of the exogenous genes in non-target tissue, French and colleagues recently described an AAV vector system employing the cardiac troponin T promoter (cTnT) (Prasad et al., 2011). AAV-9 mediated gene expression from the cTnT promoter was 640-fold greater in heart compared to liver in one week old mice. However, this transcription targeting with tissue-restricted promoters did not reduce virus accumulation or gene transfer to off-target tissue. Only the expression of the off-target gene was significantly reduced, thus deleterious side effects of viral accumulation in peripheral tissue (liver) could still persist.

These earlier successes in the rodent models provided the impetus for investigators to test the various AAV serotypes in larger animals (canine, swine). Both the minimally invasive systemic delivery approach and the invasive catheter-based coronary perfusion approach were examined. The minimally invasive approach did not yield the high level of gene transfer observed for the rodent models (Wasala et al., 2011). In newborn dogs, Yue delivered AAV via a systemic vein injection and assessed gene transfer in the heart (Yue 2008). The AAV-9 serotype resulted in minimal transduction of the heart yet significant transduction of skeletal muscle. Similarily, Bish delivered AAV-6,8, and 9 to dogs via a relatively non-invasive percutaneous transendocardial delivery approach and observed poor gene transfer to the heart with AAV 8 and 9 (Bish et al., 2008). Alternatively, gene transfer to the heart was significantly improved when the AAV was delivered by the more invasive catheter-based coronary perfusion approach. In swine, Kasper tested direct intracoronary delivery of AAV-2 and observed 8 weeks expression with no inflammatory response (Kasper et al., 2005). Similarily, Raake reported long-term expression via coronary retro-infusion using AAV-6 in heart, though transfection was also detected in liver and lung (Raake et al., 2008). In a swine model of heart failure, Hardri reported that intracoronary delivery of SERCA2a, via AAV-1, significantly improved systolic function and coronary blood flow (Hardri et al., 2010). Thus, while the AAV approach provides for long-term expression of targeted genes to the heart in the large animal models, it still requires the more invasive catheter-based approach for delivery to achieve adequate transgene efficiency. Even with the catheter-based approach, the accumulation of viral particles and transfer of genes to non-target tissue persist if the delivery is not contained within the heart.

In large animals, the highest efficiency of cardiac-specific gene transfer by viral delivery has been achieved using a closed-loop coronary recirculation strategy. White et al reported a novel surgical procedure (MCARD) that allowed for closed recirculation of AAV vectors in the cardiac circulation using cardiopulmonary bypass in sheep (White et al., 2011). This approach resulted in highly efficient, cardiac specific gene transfer using the scAAV6 vector. Similarily, Kaye and colleagues have reported a recirculation approach (V-Focus) with moderate results (Kaye et al., 2009). Coronary venous blood containing the viral vectors was recaptured from the coronary sinus with the use of a percutaneously positioned occlusive balloon recovery catheter. The captured blood, containing the viral vectors, was re-oxygenated, and returned directly to the left coronary territory via a non-occlusive catheter placed percutaneously in the left main coronary artery. At the conclusion of the recirculation period, blood continued to be removed from the coronary sinus for a short time interval to capture any remove and unsequestered virus, thereby minimizing gene transfer to non-target tissue.

2.3 The pro's and con's of the adenovirus versus adeno-associated virus

Below, we provide a summary of some of the key advantages and disadvantages of the adenovirus vs adeno-associated vector used to deliver exogenous genes to the whole heart, in vivo, via the different delivery approaches.

- While the catheter-based delivery of adenovirus requires a surgically invasive approach in rodent, compared to the non-invasive delivery of AAV (ie., delivery by simple tail vein injection), the catheter-based approach can be cardiac specific. That is, after the Adv virus is delivered to the heart via the catheter-based cross-clamp approach, unsequestered virus can be flushed from the heart before releasing the cross-clamp. Co-infection of peripheral tissue is therefore minimal. With tail vein delivery of AAV there is still co-infection of peripheral organs (liver, skeletal muscle).

- While the delivery of AAV via the tail vein in rodent models is minimally invasive, delivery of AAV in larger animals and humans still currently requires an invasive catheter-based closed-loop recirculated strategy. This is required to maximize the concentration of the virus delivered to the heart, while reducing viral accumulation and gene transfer to non-target tissue.
- An important distinction between the Adv and AAV approach relates to both how quickly and how long the delivered gene is overexpressed. The Adv_cDNA delivery provides maximum overexpresson of the protein within one week of gene transfer, compared to a gradual (1-3 mths) increase in expression via AAV_cDNA delivery. While the overexpression via Adv is relatively immediate, the overexpression is short term (2 weeks). Alternatively, protein overexpression is sustained for 3-12 months following AAV-cDNA delivery. Thus, the AAV-cDNA package provides chronic overexpression of targeted proteins, and Adv-cDNA provides acute overexpression.
- This important distinction between an acute or chronic expression predisposes the two viral packages for very different experimental applications. The immediate response of the Adv is ideal for experimental studies designed to examine the direct effects of overexpressing the targeted protein on specific biochemical, molecular, or functional responses. With AAV, any changes in biochemical, molecular, or cardiac function is in response to the gradual and long term overexpression of the targeted protein. It is difficult to define whether the observed changes with AAV_cDNA delivery are a direct response to the change in targeted protein, or if they are a secondary response due to whole organ or whole body adaptations.
- The adenovirus, Adv, is physically a much larger virus compared to the AAV. This is both good and bad. While the smaller size of the AAV enables the virus to cross the endothelial barrier with greater ease compared to the Adv, the smaller physical size of the AAV limits the length of the genome that can be packaged into the capsid. That insert capacity for the recombinant AAV is <5.2 kbases, whereas the insert capacity for the Adv is ~10 to 30 kb in length. The genome must include the inserting gene, a promoter, and a polyadenylation linker. The promoter can be as large as 1.5 kb and the polyA linker 1kb, leaving ~3.4 kb for inserting the gene in the AAV, and ~6.5 kb in the Adv. Thus, while the smaller physical size of the AAV is advantageous in terms of crossing the endothelial barrier, the larger Adv can deliver much larger genes. To circumvent the difficulty of crossing the barrier with the Adv, the use of vascular permeabilizing agents such as histamine, papaverine, substance P, low Ca^{2+} cardioplegia, and/or whole body cooling have been employed to relax the barrier and improve viral delivery.
- The Adv can be used to transfer exogenous genes to the heart multiple times. The AAV can only be used once due to an autoimmune response to the virus.
- The synthesis of the adenovirus-cDNA package is much easier than the AAV-cDNA package. The insertion of the cDNA into the Adv vector and the subsequent amplification of the virus is now routine, available thru multiple vendors and core facilities, and can be amplified in standard laboratories. Amplification via cell-to-cell transmission in HEK 293 cells with the Adv enables large-scale concentrations (10^{13}

vp/ml) and volumes. On the other hand, AAV production requires vector quantities which are not easily produced in laboratory or most research-grade vector core facilities. The most established methods for producing AAV use adherent HEK 293 cells chemically co-transfected with plasmids encoding the necessary virus proteins (Kotin, 2011). However, the absence of cell-to-cell transmission limits AAV production to cells initially transfected with plasmid DNA, thereby limiting the production titer and volume (10^{10} vp/ml at best).

- The Adv induces an inflammatory response in heart after 4-5 days. The inflammatory response is minimal with AAV with the first treatment.
- While some of the serotypes of AAV do show specificity for heart, infection of non-target tissue presists. To improve cardiac specific expression of the protein, cardiac promoters are used instead of the ubiquitously strong CMV promoter (AAV9 with cardiac troponin T promoter cTnT; Prasad et al., 2011). While this does reduce the expression of the gene in non-target tissue, expression in the heart is also attenuated without the strong CMV promoter. Furthermore, while the expression of the gene in non-target tissue is reduced by using the cardiac-specific promoters, the accumulation of viral particles in non-target tissue (liver) is unchanged.

3. Two catheter-based methods for adenoviral gene delivery to rat heart, in vivo

3.1 The conventional catheter-based, cross-clamp method

The conventional open-chest cross-clamp approach has been described extensively in previous reports (Miyamoto et al., 2000; Del Monte et al., 2001, 2002). In brief, the chest was entered by a median sternotomy and a 22-gauge catheter containing 100 ml of adenoviral solution was advanced from the apex of the left ventricle to the aortic root. The aorta and pulmonary arteries were clamped distal to the site of the catheter and the viral solution (~$2x10^{12}$ vp/ml) was injected (high pressure). The clamp was maintained for 30 seconds. Only those hearts demonstrating the hallmark 'blanching', or whitening, during viral injection were maintained post-operatively for assessment of infection.

3.2 The catheter-based, retrograde perfusion method

Our advancement enables a completely isolated heart to be continuously retrograde perfused, in vivo, thereby (a) providing a blood-free pretreatment period with endothelial barrier relaxation agents (ie., calcium free Tyrode solution) prior to the delivery of the viral solution, and (b) enabling unsequestered virus to be flushed from the heart prior to releasing the cross-clamp, thereby eliminating gene transfer and viral accumulation in non-target organs (O'Donnell et al., 2005, 2006).

Figure 2 illustrates the scheme of the catheter-based approach for the retrograde perfusion of the isolated heart, in vivo. In brief, adult male Sprague-Dawley rats (350 g) were anesthetized (isoflurane), intubated, and placed on an ice pad to cool the core body temperature to 30°C. While the temperature lowered, the chest was opened from the right side at the second or third intercostal space. The pericardium was opened and 4-0 silk was sutured at the apex of the heart (see Figure 2). The suture was used to control handling / positioning of the heart. A 20-gauge catheter was inserted through the apex into the left ventricle. The tip of the catheter was advanced to the aortic root. Placement of the tip was verified by observing the tip through the wall of the ascending aorta. The catheter was connected to tubing for delivery of perfusate solution and adenovirus via a peristaltic pump. The catheter was tied to the 4–0 suture that was placed at the apex of the heart. This kept the catheter from sliding out of position during the perfusion protocol.

The heart was externalized from the rib cage and all vessels leading to and from the heart (superior/inferior vena cava, pulmonary artery/vein, and ascending aorta) were occluded simultaneously with a single cross-clamp. The clamp was distal to the catheter positioned in the aortic root. A 24-gauge catheter was inserted into the right ventricle. This catheter provided a path for perfusate efflux from the heart. Next, the heart was retrograde perfused, in vivo, with well oxygenated calcium-free tyrode solution for 7.5 min via the catheter positioned in the aortic root. The perfusate flow rate was 3–30 ml/min, and the efflux was discarded. Following this permeability treatment phase with calcium free buffer, the perfusion was stopped and the adenovirus was injected thru the perfusion catheter (0.2 ml of AdV.cmv.SERCA1 in PBS; 10^{12} viral particles/ml). Excess solution dripped from the efflux catheter. This allowed the adenovirus to circulate down the coronaries. Next, the efflux catheter positioned in the right ventricle was removed, and an additional 0.5 ml/kg of adenovirus (~0.2 ml) was delivered to the aortic root (1 sec) at a peak pressure of 300 ± 100 mmHg. After 90 s, catheters were positioned in the right and left ventricles, and unsequestered virus was flushed from the heart with well oxygenated Krebs buffer containing calcium delivered through the perfusion line. This washout period with buffer containing Ca^{2+} (1.5 mM) aided in contractile recovery. The chest was then closed, air was evacuated, and the body was warmed to 37°C. Once the animal could breath independently, the rat was moved to an oxygen chamber until it recovered from the anesthesia (1 h). After 2-3 days, hearts were excised for the analysis of SERCA expression (Western blots), functional measurements (in vivo and ex vivo), and metabolic measurement (^{31}P and ^{13}C NMR experiments).

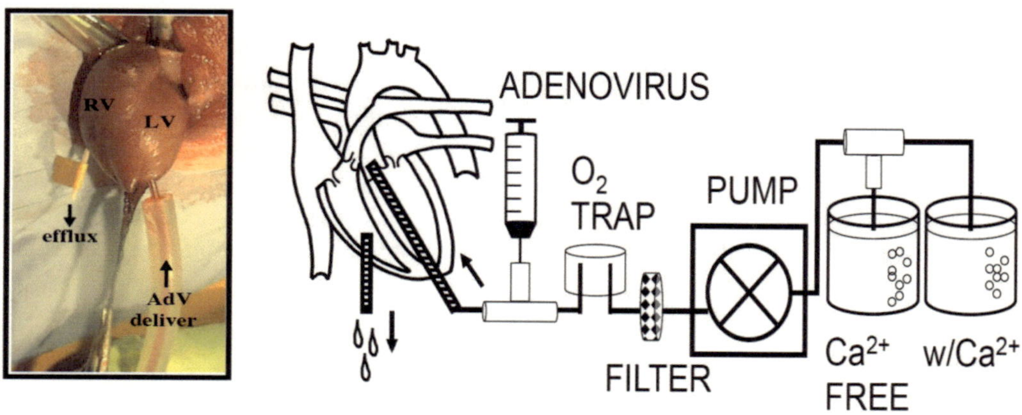

Fig. 2. Photo of a rat heart instrumented for catheter-based delivery of adenovirus into the aortic root. The hearts were completely isolated in vivo and retrograde perfused with calcium free Tyrode solution for 7.5 minutes before a single bolus of Adv.cmv.LacZ (10^{12} vp/ml in 400 ml PBS) was delivered into the aortic root. A catheter positioned in the aortic root provided the route for Adv delivery. A second catheter in the right ventricle provided a route for perfusate efflux during the retrograde perfusion period. (Reprinted from O'Donnell et al., 2006)

We noted several key methodological nuances that influenced the level of infection in the heart. First, during viral injection, no tension could be put on the heart. If the heart was stretched or compressed during injection of the virus, infection was focus to the atria and right ventricle, suggesting compromised coronary perfusion. In addition, the heart did not perfuse properly if the left ventricle filled with perfusate during the isolation. If the left ventricle appeared to hyperextend during perfusion, a second catheter was inserted into the left ventricle to reduce intraventricular pressure. We also noted an important limitation with the preparation of the virus. Viral amplifications taken out past five passages yielded the very high titers required; however, the expression of LacZ was reduced in the infected heart. This is consistent with the known rearrangement of the Ad5.LacZ vector at the sixth passage. For this reason, we always started with first-generation virus and stopped the amplification at the fifth passage.

Survival rates. The survival rate following this invasive procedure is on the order of 80-100% in healthy animals. It depends largely on the skill of the surgeon. This is clearly a non-trivial procedure. We find it takes 1-3 months of weekly practice for a previously untrained technician to master the skills required for any type of open-chest survival surgery (ie., aortic banding or catheter based viral_cDNA delivery). In addition, there is a risk that a novice surgeon can damage the aortic valve when the catheter is inserted through the apex of the heart and advance to the aortic root (as detected by echocardiograms). Survival rates for rats in early stages of decompensated left ventricular heart failure (10-12 weeks post banding) is >70% following the surgical procedure. Rats do not survive this procedure, or any open-chest surgical procedure, if performed at end-stage heart failure (>20 weeks post-banding).

3.3 Reporter gene considerations

Reporter genes are used to assess the efficiency of gene delivery by the various delivery approaches and delivery vectors. Two of the more common reporter genes include GFP and LacZ (β-Gal). GFP has not always been favored as a reporter gene for studies of gene transfer to the heart, in part because it can be difficult to distinguish authentic GFP fluorescence above endogenous background autofluorescene (Prasad et al., 2011). This is illustrated in Figure 3. This figure shows high regions of fluorescence which could be interpreted as areas of GFP expression. However, this is actually background autofluorescene from a section of untreated heart which had not been uniformly sliced and mounted on the slide.

The reporter gene, LacZ, is an attractive alternative. Following vector delivery of cDNA for LacZ, the efficiency of LacZ gene transfer is assessed after X-Gal staining of the whole heart or individual slices of the heart cross-section. Positive cells for Lac Z expression turn blue with X-Gal staining. In the cross-sectional preparations, the efficiency of gene transfer is calculated as the number of blue cells relative to the total number of cells. In whole heart staining, the heart is first fixed, stained, and digested (collagenase) by retrograde perfusion (O'Donnell et al., 2005, 2006). Then, the efficiency of gene transfer is measured in the isolated cell preparation as the fraction of blue cells expressing LacZ.

The LacZ approach does require careful interpretation of the results. First, some organs do have a low level of endogenous LacZ expression. It is not always clear if this endogenous signal increases in response to the disease model or the surgical intervention of gene transfer. Therefore, it is important to confirm the relative change in endogenous signal in sham-operated animals and disease models without viral gene transfer. In the case of the aortic-banded pressure-overloaded rat model of cardiac hypertrophy, the change in endogenous LacZ signal is minimal in the heart (O'Donnell et al., 2008). Secondly, the expression of LacZ can be assessed by a colorimetric assay for the increase in blue signal from tissue samples. However, the colorimetric approach is not a direct measure of the efficiency of gene transfer. While it is a useful tool to measure a relative change in the level of LacZ expression, the actual RLU reading (relative light units) provides no insight for the number, or efficiency, of cells infected. Finally, care must be taken in reporting the efficiency of LacZ gene transfer by photographic illustration. As illustrated in Figure 3, an image which shows only a small region of heart for LacZ expression is not representative of the whole heart, and it does not properly reflect the efficiency of transfer. Nevertheless, when properly performed, the LacZ reporter gene is an excellent and widely used tool to assess and compare the efficiency of gene transfer by various delivery techniques.

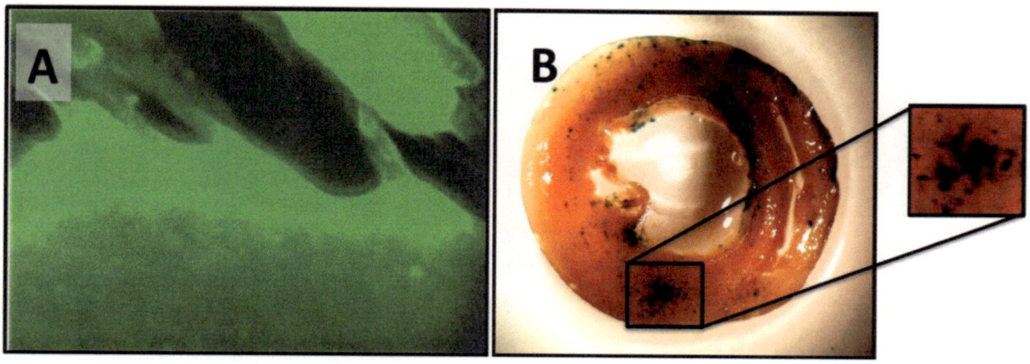

Fig. 3. Adenoviral gene transfer for the reporter gene (A) GFP and (B) LacZ in heart by the conventional cross-clamp technique. Interpretation of reporter gene data can often be misleading. While there is significant green fluorescence visible in a section of heart on the left, this figure is actually background fluorescence. The heart was not infected with Adv.cmv.GFP. This section of heart was not evenly sliced and mounted on the slide, thereby accounting for regions of greater GFP expression. The heart on the right was indeed infected with Adv.cmv.LacZ via the conventional cross-clamp approach. While the full cross-section indicates that the efficiency of transfer was low (ie., dark blue cells), the selected inset shown on the right inappropriately suggests that the transfection was quite good.

3.4 Efficiency of gene transfer in heart

Figure 4 shows the extent of LacZ expression, following X-Gal staining, through multiple cross-sections of a heart 72 h after Ad.cmv.LacZ delivery to the heart, in vivo. The heart was isolated *in vivo* and retrograde perfused for 7.5min with calcium-free Tyrode solution before delivery of a single bolus of PBS containing adenovirus (Ad.cmv.LacZ, 400 ml, 10^{12} pfu/ml in PBS). Transfected hearts were also digested (collagenase) after X-Gal staining, and the efficiency of gene transfer was assessed by blue cell counts. Importantly, this strategy resulted in significant and global gene transfer to the whole heart. The efficiency of gene transfer was 58 ± 11%.

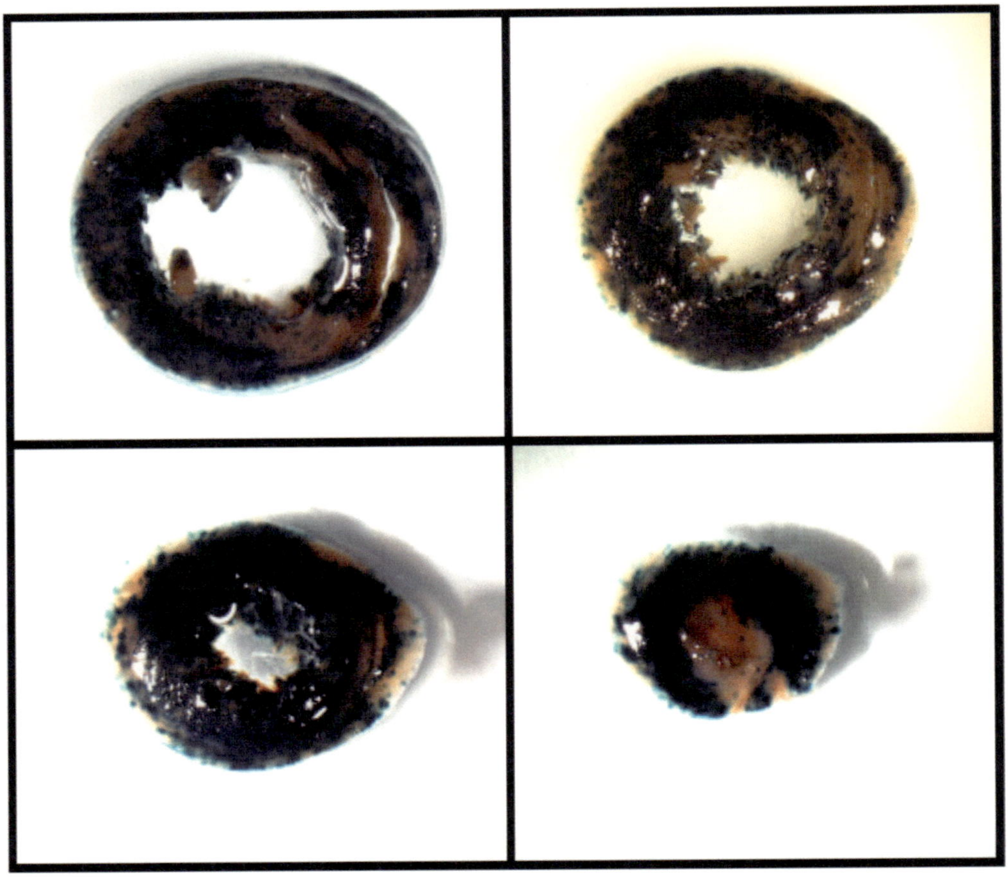

Fig. 4. Cross sections of heart stained (X-Gal) for LacZ expression following gene transfer *in vivo* by the isolated heart perfusion approach. The heart was completed isolated *in vivo* and retrograde perfused with calcium free Tyrode solution for 7.5 minutes before a single bolus of Adv.cmv.LacZ (10^{12} vp/ml in 400 ml PBS) was delivered into the aortic root. The blue regions demonstrate cells expressing the transferred gene. The efficiency of gene transfer to the heart was 58 ± 11 %. (Reprinted from O'Donnell et al., 2005)

3.5 Gene transfer to non-target organs

We assessed the level of Ad.cmv.LacZ infection in heart, liver, lung, and skeletal muscle based on a colorimetric RLU assay quantifying β-Gal activity. The intent was to determine if flushing unsequesterd virus from the heart, prior to removing the cross-clamp, reduced infection of peripheral tissue compared to the conventional cross-clamp approach. The results are shown in Figure 5. In liver, β-Gal activity was dramatically reduced compared to the conventional cross-clamp approach. Infection of lung and muscle was nearly undetectable. Conversely, the level of β-Gal activity in the heart (ie., post gene transfer) was 4–10 times greater by the isolated, retrograde perfusion approach compared to the conventional cross-clamp approach. The reduction in the infection of peripheral organs is consistent with having flushed all unsequestered virus from the heart prior to releasing the cross-clamp.

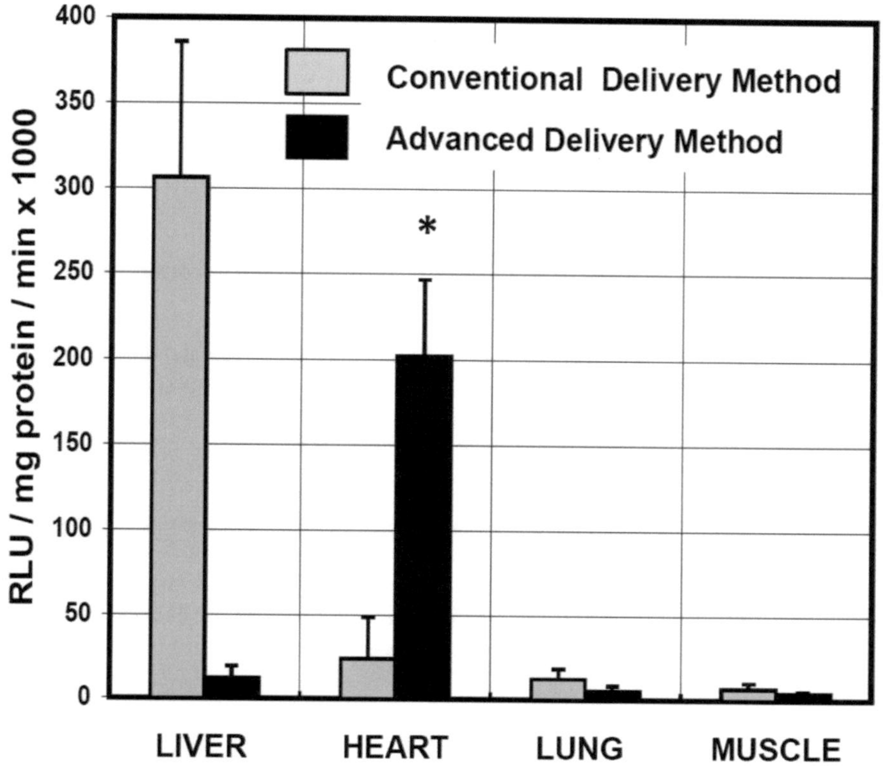

Fig. 5. The solid gray bars illustrate the level of in vivo gene transfer by a conventional aorta/pulmonary artery cross-clamp technique. Infection by our isolated, retrograde perfusion approach is shown in black. The conventional method results in significant infection of the liver and peripheral tissue. Our scheme results in significantly greater gene transfer to the heart while reducing liver infection dramatically. (Reprinted from O'Donnell et al., 2005)

4. SERCA gene therapy for heart failure: Good or bad?

The changes in intracellular Ca2+□ handling reported for the failing myocardium have been linked to the sarco(endo)plasmic reticulum Ca2+-ATPase (SERCA) (Gwathmey et al., 1987). Calcium uptake into the sarcoplasmic reticulum (SR) by SERCA determines the rate of calcium removal for relaxation, the SR calcium content, and calcium released for contractions (Periasamy et al., 2001). In the failing heart, it has been proposed that SERCA contributes to reduced contractility and relaxation as the activity and number of these calcium transporters are reduced and calcium transients are blunted and slow to decay (Gwathmey et al., 1987; Chang et al., 1996; Miyamoto et al., 2000).

There is overwhelming evidence that the overexpression of SERCA2a in the failing myocardium from both animal models and humans leads to enhance cardiac function and improved survival (review Gwathmey et al., 2011). Surprisingly, we found the overexpression of the SERCA1 isoform actually compromised cardiac performance, in vivo (O'Donnell et al., 2008). Our finding was recently supported by a second report (heart failure model in SERCA2a transgenic mice) (Pinz et al., 2011). These opposing results raise concerns regarding the safety of the current translational clinical studies in human (Hajjar et al., 2008; Jaski et al., 2009; Gwathmey et al., 2011). Here, we will briefly highlight the progression of the earlier studies in whole heart and isolated cardiomyocytes which support the therapeutic strategy. We will discuss the opposing results from our study and the recent transgenic mouse study, and we will provide some considerations which may account for the discrepany between reports. The controversy of this therapeutic strategy as it relates to the stage and model of the disease is also discussed in a recent commentary by Sipido and Bangheluwe (Sipido et al., 2010).

4.1 Positive outcome with SERCA in isolated cardiomyocytes from human

Indeed, a number of groups have reported that the overexpression of either the isoform for SERCA2a or SERCA1 in isolated cardiomyocytes lead to enhanced cell shortening, and accelerated uptake of calcium by the sarcoplasmic reticulum. In non-treated myocytes isolated from patients with end-stage heart failure, the calcium transient is blunted and the sequestration of calcium slowed (Gwathmey et al., 1987). If this is truly a maladaptive alternation, and not compensatory, then it is reasonable to hypothesized that increasing the rate of calcium sequestration may enhance the relaxation rate. Indeed, Del Monte et al demonstrated that the transfer of SERCA2a cDNA into isolated cardiomyocytes from failing human hearts restored contractile function (Del Monte et al., 1999). Similarily, Weisser-Thomas provided further evidence that the overexpression of the SERCA1 isoform in isolated cardiomyocytes from patients in heart failure also had beneficial effects (Weisser-Thomas et al., 2005).

4.2 Positive outcome with SERCA2a in whole heart models of heart failure

The encouraging results from the isolated cardiomyocyte studies provided the impetus to examine the effects in animal models of heart failure. Hajjar subsequently developed the catheter-based cross-clamp approach for the delivery of genes to rat heart in vivo (Del Monte et al., 2002). His group demonstrated that the overexpression of the SERCA2a isoform in the aortic-banded rat model of left-ventricular function improved cardiac function and survival (Miyamoto et al., 2000; Del Monte et al., 2001). The strategy was then performed in a larger animal model (sheep) with heart failure induced by fast pacing (Byrne et al., 2008). Results were similarly encouraging. These early studies in animals models of cardiac disease have now been translated to clinical trials, and results from recent early phase clinical trials in humans find fewer episodic events and improvement in multiple end-points (such as left ventricular end-systolic volume, walking tests, oxygen consumption) with no adverse events, following delivery of SERCA2a via AAV-1 via a catheter based approach (Hajjar et al., 2008; Jaski et al., 2009; Gwathmey et al., 2011). However, LV ejection fraction did not increase appreciably with any of the three AAV_SERCA2a doses examined (Jessup et al., 2011). Two other clinical trials targeting SERCA2a are currently enrolling patients. The trials are being conducted in the United Kingdom and the Institut of Cardiology Pitié-Salpêtrière, Paris, France, with the primary objective to investigate the impact of AAV6- CMV-SERCA2a on cardiac remodeling parameters in patients with severe heart failure.

4.3 Negative outcome with SERCA1a in whole heart models of heart failure

In our study, Ad.cmv.LacZ, Ad.cmv.SERCA1, or PBS was delivered, in vivo, to aortic banded (10-12 wks) and sham operated Sprague Dawley rats by our catheter-based perfusion technique described above. Compared to the cardiac isoform (SERCA2a) SERCA1 is not regulated by phospholamban, and has a higher activity with a two-fold greater calcium uptake relative to SERCA2a. SERCA1 is also more resistant to oxidative stress and acidosis.

The subset of banded and sham rats receiving Adv.cmv.LacZ (10^{12} viral particles/ml), were used here to confirm the efficiency of gene transfer in the disease model. X-Gal staining for LacZ gene transfer revealed significant and heterogeneously expression throughout both the sham and banded hearts 48-72 hrs following Ad.cmv.LacZ delivery, similar to the level of overexpression illustrated in figure 4. Importantly, there were no "false positives" for endogenous LacZ expression in hearts as a consequence of microinfarctions formed during the intracoronary infusion as previously speculated by Wright et al (Wright et al., 1998).

Western blot analysis for SERCA2a, SERCA1, and calsequestrin are shown in Figure 6 for sham and banded hearts receiving Ad.cmv.SERCA1. In the 10-12 week banded and sham groups receiving the PBS vehicle without adenovirus, SERCA2a expression was similar between groups. SERCA2a levels are not expected to drop until late-stage failure in the rat model (Arai et al., 1996). Importantly, in the banded and sham groups receiving the Adv.cmv.SERCA1, SERCA1 protein was significantly overexpressed. Densitometry analysis of Coomassie blue stained gels indicated that the total SERCA content increased by 34 ± 15% in both banded and sham hearts, and endogenous SERCA2a expression levels were unaffected. Indeed, this level of expression is lower than the level reported for the SERCA1 transgenic mouse model and our own earlier cardiomyocyte data (Cavagna et al., 2000; Loukianov et al., 1998). In transgenic mice expressing SERCA1, total SERCA levels increased by 2.5-fold and endogenous SERCA2a expression were reduced by 50%(Huke et al., 2002; Lalli et al., 2001; Loukianov et al., 1998). In cardiomyocytes, total SERCA levels increased by 3 fold and SERCA2a dropped by 50%. The higher level of gene transfer in isolated cardiomyocytes is consistent with a much higher multiplicity of infection (MOI). In cardiomyocyte the MOI is typically 2 to 10 vp/cell (O'Donnell et al., 2001). In the intact heart, the MOI is typically <0.5 at best (ie., 50% efficiency) (O'Donnell et al., 2008). Nevertheless, a contractile response was still elicited both in vivo and ex vivo following the catheter-based delivery of SERCA1 to whole hearts.

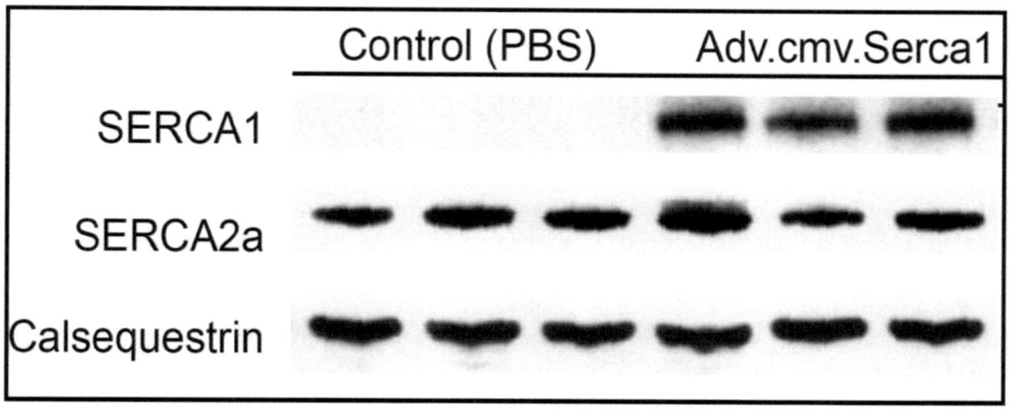

Fig. 6. Western blot data for SERCA1, SERCA2a, and calsequestrin expression following Adv.cmv.SERCA1 gene transfer or PBS (control) in rat heart. Densitometry analysis of Coomassie blue stained gels indicated that the total SERCA content increased by 34 ± 15% with adenoviral transfer of SERCA1 cDNA. Endogenous SERCA2a expression levels were unaffected. (Reprinted from O'Donnell et al., 2009)

Hemodynmic consequences of SERCA1 overexpression. The echocardiographic measurements made 48–72 h after PBS delivery or adenoviral gene delivery of SERCA1 cDNA in both sham and banded LVH rat hearts are listed in Table 1. There were no significant differences between sham groups receiving either catheter-based delivery of PBS or Ad.cmv.SERCA1. LV dimensions were similar, as were LV wall thickness and fractional shortening. After 10 wk of aortic banding, LVH_PBS animals showed echocardiographic signs of LVH relative to the SHM_PBS group, as expected, including a significant increase in the LV systolic dimension and a decrease in fractional shortening. Importantly, these parameters were not reverse with SERCA1 treatment. LV diastolic and systolic dimensions actually increased 10–15%, whereas fractional shortening was reduced by an additional 17%. This change indicates further LV remodeling with SERCA1 expression in failing hearts in this study. A decrease in the LV posterior wall systole dimension (LVPWS) in the SERCA1 treated LVH group (LVH_SR1) was also measured, and is consistent with further dilation. Importantly, this data for the overexpression of SERCA1 challenges the existing hemodynamic / functional data for the overexpression of SERCA2a in this rat model of left ventricular hypertrophy (Miyamoto et al., 2000; Del Monte et al., 2001). Whether this is linked to the specific isoform of SERCA is unclear, and it raises a cautionary flag regarding the current clinical trails.

	Heart/body (g/kg)	Heart rate (bpm)	LVDd (mm)	LVSd (mm)	FS (%)	Vcf (circ/s)	LVPWD (mm)	LVPWS (mm)
SHM_PBS (n=4)	6.20	335 ± 25	8.2 ± 0.9	4.8 ± 0.4	40.6 ± 5.7	0.027 ± 0.005	1.3 ± 0.4	2.4 ± 0.3
SHM_SR1 (n=7)	6.19	334 ± 36	8.5 ± 0.8	5.2 ± 0.9	38.9 ± 5.6	0.026 ± 0.003	1.2 ± 0.2	2.2 ± 0.3
LVH_PBS (n=6)	9.22*	332 ± 20	8.5 ± 0.1	5.9 ± 0.1*	30.5 ± 4.2*	0.025 ± 0.003	1.4 ± 0.1	2.3 ± 0.1
LVH_SR1 (n=7)	9.25†	320 ± 27	9.1 ± 0.1†	6.8 ± 0.1†§	25.3 ± 5.3†	0.020 ± 0.004§	1.3 ± 0.1	2.0 ± 0.1

Table 1. LVDd indicates LV diastole dimension; LVSd, LV systole dimension; FS, fractional shortening; Vcf, velocity of circumferential shortening; LVPWD, LV posterior wall diastole dimension; LVPWS, LV posterior wall systole dimension. *P<0.05 LVH_PBS vs SHM_PBS or SHM_SR1; †P<0.05 LVH_SR1 vs SHM_PBS or SHM_SR1; §P<0.05 LVH_SR1 vs LVH_PBS. (Reprinted from O'Donnell et al., 2008)

Following the in vivo echocardiography measurements, hearts were excised, retrograde perfused, and both cardiac function and metabolic activity were assessed. The ex vivo data revealed a very different functional response to SERCA1 overexpression compared to in vivo data. In excised SHM hearts overexpressing SERCA1, there was a modest increase in RPP yet a profound positive impact on contractility rates (±dP/d*t*). HR was unaffected. The accelerated relaxation (-dP/d*t*) is consistent with a faster removal of calcium from the cytosol as the number of SERCA pumps are overexpressed. These results compared favorably with functional data reported for isolated, work-performing hearts from SERCA1 transgenic mice (Huke et al., 2002). Huke and colleagues also reported a 20% increase in LVDP, whereas □±dP/d*t* nearly doubled, and HR was unchanged. However, much like our own in vivo data, they did not find dramatic changes in vivo (Huke et al., 2002). They suggested that the differences between *ex vivo* and *in vivo* data reflect the presence of *in vivo* compensatory mechanisms that "normalize" cardiac function in transgenic mice.

For the excised LVH hearts overexpressing SERCA1, RPP recovered to normal levels at baseline. However, the relaxation rate (-dP/d*t*) and LVDP did not improve with treatment. Instead, the improvement in the RPP was linked to a 20% increase in HR. These hearts were not paced. This finding was unexpected and suggests a physiological link between SERCA function and HR regulation. It is unclear to what extent SERCA influences the electrical excitability and repolarization of cardiomyocytes or potentially the neurons that innervate the heart. It was also unexpected that the overexpression of SERCA1 in the LVH group did not lead to enhanced LVDP or relaxation rates in isolated hearts. We originally hypothesized that the overexpression of SERCA1 would lead to a faster calcium uptake by the SR, thereby accelerating relaxation and potentiating LVDP as seen in SERCA1 overexpressing shams. However, our finding is more consistent with the hypothesis that calcium sequestration by the SR may not be the limiting factor affecting LVDP and relaxation in the failing heart.

Experimental summary. Although previous cardiomyocyte data and non- hypertrophic transgenic mouse models have revealed important and positive functional and metabolic responses to SERCA1 isoform overexpression, this study extended those earlier findings to include the intact functioning hypertrophic heart expressing SERCA1 under both in vivo and ex vivo conditions. In support of previous work, we found that the overexpression of SERCA1 in isolated heart preparations resulted in enhanced function and sustained energy potentials. At higher workloads, SERCA1 expression influenced energy metabolism by increasing glucose oxidation, thereby potentially making overall energy production more efficient. However, under the fully loaded in vivo condition, function was not affected in healthy hearts overexpressing SERCA1 at basal workloads, and hypertrophic hearts revealed depressed function with SERCA1 expression. Further investigation is required to determine if this is a consequence of whole body compensatory mechanisms or a limitation in the competitive handling of calcium between the SR versus myofilaments.

4.4 Negative outcome with SERCA2a transgenic mice in heart failure

Pinz examined the effects of SERCA2a overexpresion on cardiac performance and energetic costs in left ventricular hypertrophy transgenic mouse model (Pinz et al., 2011). Mouse hearts were isolated and perfused from wild-type and transgenic mice overexpressing the cardiac isoform of SERCA2a, 8 weeks after ascending aortic-banding (left ventricular hypertrophy). SERCA2a mRNA and protein levels were decreased more than 50% in banded wild-type hearts compared to wild-type shams. The expression of SERCA2a mRNA and protein levels in the transgenic hypertrophic group was normalized compare to the wild-type hearts. They found that overexpressing SERCA2a enhanced myocardial contraction and relaxation in normal transgenic mouse hearts during inotropic stimulation with isoproterenol, and energy comsumption was proportionate to contractile function. However, the increased amount of SERCA2a in hypertrophied hearts was not sufficient to support or increase contractile function of these hearts above the level achieved by hypertrophied wild-type hearts. These results indicated that the positive effect of overexpressing SERCA2a on myocardial contractiliy was not maintined in hypertrophic hearts. Furthermore, despite the finding of greater energy efficency with higher levels of SERCA2a in normal transgenic hearts, they did not find a beneficial energetic effect in hypertrophied hearts overexpressing SERCA2a. Instead, they observed a downward shift in the relationship between contractile force and free energy available from ATP hydrolysis in hypertrophied transgenic hearts when compared with sham transgenics, suggesting that energy supply may be a limiting factor for the benefit of SERCA2a overexpression in hypertrophied hearts. Taken together, they concluded that the strategy of increasing SERCA activity may not be effective in all models and/or stages of cardiac dysfunction (Pinz et al., 2011).

4.5 Potential mechanisms for the discrepancies between reports

4.5.1 Dose-response effects

Teucher and colleaques examined the effects of different levels of SERCA1a expression on contractility and Ca^{2+} cycling in isolated cardiomyocytes in heart of rabbit transfected at different multiplicities of infection (Teucher et al., 2004). They examined whether increased SERCA1a expression levels enhanced myocyte contractility in a gene-dose-dependent manner. At a MOI 10 vp/cell, myocytes expressing SERCA1a (versus Ad-LacZ controls) revealed enhanced SR Ca^{2+}□ uptake, relaxation rates, SR Ca^{2+}□content, isotonic shortening, and Ca^{2+} transient amplitude. At higher SERCA expression levels (MOI 50), myocytes exhibited further increases in SR Ca^{2+}□uptake, relaxation rate, and SR Ca^{2+}□content but showed depressed contraction amplitude and no Ca2+□transient enhancement versus control. They concluded that high SERCA activity causes a paradoxical decrease in contractile activation because of greater Ca2+□removal from the cytosol, and that the use of SERCA1a for gene therapy in heart failure requires careful control of transfection efficiency and induced expression levels.

4.5.2 Maladaptive myofilament effects

In our study described above, it was unexpected that the overexpression of SERCA1 in the LVH group did not lead to enhanced LVDP or relaxation rates in isolated hearts. We originally hypothesized that the overexpression of SERCA1 would lead to a faster calcium uptake by the SR, thereby accelerating relaxation and potentiating LVDP. Our finding is more consistent with the hypothesis that calcium sequestration by the SR may not be the limiting factor affecting LVDP and relaxation in the failing heart (Janssen et al., 2002; Perez et al., 1999). In brief, if reuptake of Ca2□ becomes too fast, the cytoplasmic calcium concentration near the myofilaments will decline rapidly, preventing the appropriate activation of myofilaments and hindering adequate force development (Janssen et al., 2002; Teucher et al., 2004). Thus, the SR competes with troponin C for calcium binding (Hiranandani et al., 2007; Janssen et al., 2002; Loukianov et al., 1998; Teucher et al., 2004). In heart failure, the calcium sensitivity of myofilaments is altered in both human and rodent models (Marston et al., 2008). A potential adverse effect of increasing calcium sensitivity is slowed relaxation and diastolic dysfunction (MacGowan, 2005). If myofilament properties are limiting the relaxation rate and force development in heart failure, the overexpression of SERCA would be competitive and deleterious.

In addition, the majority of studies that concluded that calcium sequestration limited the relaxation rate were performed in isolated cardiomyocytes. Under such unloaded conditions, cross-bridges cycle much faster than loaded cross-bridges, and the sequestration rate by the SR may indeed limit cytosolic calcium decline (Janssen et al., 2007). However, under loaded conditions, relaxation of the myocardium may be more closely linked to myofilment properties (Janssen et al., 2002, 2007). Indeed, Teucher and colleagues (2004) also reported that moderate SERCA1 gene transfer and expression improved contractility and Ca^{2+} cycling in cardiomyocytes. However, higher SERCA1 expression levels impaired myocyte shortening because of higher SERCA activity and Ca^{2+} buffering. Vangheluwe et al. (2006) also demonstrated that replacement of the SERCA2a isoform with SERCA2b, an isoform with increased Ca^{2+} affinity, led to severe cardiac hypertrophy, stress intolerance, and a reduced life span in transgenic mice.

4.5.3 Animal model effects (ie., early vs late stage heart failure)

The discrepancy between the results of our study and the early rat studies may be related to the stage of heart failure model examined. In the earlier work, the effects of SERCA2a overexpression were examined in the aortic-banded rat model at a late stage of heart failure (Miyamoto et al., 2000; Del Monte et al., 2001). At this late stage of decompensated heart failure, endogenous SERCA2a content is significantly reduced in untreated hearts, and the overexpression treatment normalized SERCA2a content and reportedly had beneficial effects on cardiac function. Alternatively, we examined the consequences of SERCA overexpression at an earlier deompensated stage (10-12 weeks post-banding) of the disease in rat (O'Donnell et al., 2008). At this stage, endogenous SERCA2a expression was not reduced, and the overexpression of SERCA was deleterious. However, this argument is not supported by the SERCA2a transgenic mouse model of heart failure (Pinz et al., 2011). The transgenic mouse study was also performed at a stage of disease progression where SERCA2a mRNA and protein levels were reduced by 50%, consistent with the earlier rat study. Unlike the rat studies, normalization of protein levels in the transgenic heart failure group did not improve cardiac performance. Therefore, the opposing results of the earlier SERCA2a studies in the rat compared to our study (and transgenic mouse) study remains unresolved.

4.5.4 Problems selecting a proper control gene

There is no ideal vector to use as a control group. The control groups could receive an empty adenovirus (which is not actually empty), a bolus of PBS, or adenovirus carrying cDNA for GFP, LacZ, or scrambled cDNA. With any of the adenoviral packages, there is foreign DNA inserted into the cells, and the cells will need to deal with this foreign nucleotide and subsequent protein expressed. Our group, and others (Weisser-Thomas et al., 2005) have noted that these adenoviral "controls" do affect function relative to non-treated tissue (ie, PBS treatment). Therefore, it is not always clear if the gene of interest (ie., SERCA2a) altered baseline cardiac function, or if the control group (ie., GFP, scrambled cDNA, etc) altered baseline function. The earlier studies used βGal cDNA as the control gene in their studies (Del Monte et al., 2001), and our group used a virus free PBS control group.

5. Conclusions

There were an overwhelming number of laboratories examining the new and exciting adenoviral gene therapy strategies in the 1990's. With any new breakthrough, a number of hurdles emerged and the immediate reality of the approach did not live up to the promise. Most groups moved onto the next great thing (ie., stem cells). Some groups persevered with the viral approach, and focused their efforts on resolving the limitations. Today, we have a far greater understanding of this approach, and we are closer to the promise of this application in human. The current state-of-art approach for human application includes the use of AAV vectors delivered to the heart in a catheter-based, isolated, recirculation path. The AAV vector provides for long-term protein overexpression with minimal inflammatory or toxic effects. A number of different AAV serotypes and gene promoters are now being examined to improve targeting the gene delivery to the heart with the hope of one day simply injecting the viral package into the circulatory system. Until then, the catheter-based delivery of the viral package to the heart is required to optimize gene transfer to the heart, while reducing the accumulation of viral particles and gene transfer to non-target organs in human.

Not only is the development of this novel technology important for treatment of heart disease in humans, it is also a powerful tool for elucidating the molecular basis of cardiovascular diseases. Indeed, the results of these basic science studies in rat and mouse steer us toward the proper gene selection for disease treatments in humans. For these studies, the delivery of the exogenous genes to a completely isolated heart, in vivo, via a catheter-based approach, is required to maximize gene transfer in heart and eliminate viral accumulation and gene transfer to non-target tissue. Unlike the human treatment strategies with the AAV, we argue that the adenoviral vector Adv still provides considerable advantages for molecular based studies. The Adv vector is easy to synthesize in any lab, it provides very robust gene transfer compared to AAV, large genes can be packaged in the virus, and the overexpression of the transfer gene is maximal within 3-4 days (prior to the inflammatory response). As opposed to the chronic AAV and transgenic models, this acute response enables the scientist to directly assess the affects of protein overexpression (or silencing) on molecular processes, cardiac function, and survival.

6. Acknowledgement

This work was supported by a research grant from National Heart, Lung, and Blood Institutes Grants R01 HL-079415 (J.M. O'Donnell).

7. References

Arai M, Suzuki, Tadashi, Nagai R. Sarcoplasmic reticulum genes are up regulated in mild cardiac hypertrophy but down regulated in severe cardiac hypertrophy induced by pressure overload. *J Mol Cell Cardiol* 28: 1583– 1590, 1996.

Aikawa R, et al. Cardiomyocyte-specific gene expression following recombinant adeno-associated viral vector transduction. *J Biol Chem*. 2002. 21: 18979-18985.

Barr E, Carroll J, Kalynych AM, Tripathy SK, Kozarsky K, Wilson JM, & Leiden JM. Efficient catheter-mediated gene transfer into the heart using replication-defective adenovirus, *Gene Therapy*, 1994, 1(1), 51-8.

Bish LT, Morine K, Sleeper MM, et al. Adeno-associated virus (AAV) serotype 9 provides global cardiac gene transfer superior to AAV1, AAV6, AAV7, and AAV8 in the mouse and rat. Hum Gene Ther 2008; 19: 1359-1368.

Bish LT, Sleeper MM, Brainard B, et al. Percutaneous transendocardial delivery of self-complementary adeno-associated virus 6 achieves global cardiac gene transfer in canines. Mol Ther 2008; 16: 1953-1959.

Blankinship MJ, et al. Efficient transduction of skeletal muscle using vectors based on adeno-associated virus serotype 6. *Molecul Ther.* 2004. 10(4): 671678.

Byrne MJ, Power JM, Preovolos A, Mariani JA, Hajjar RJ, Kaye DM. Recirculating cardiac delivery of AAV2/1SERCA2a improves myocardial function in an experimental model of heart failure in large animals. Gene Ther. 2008 Dec;15(23):1550-7.

Cavagna M, O'Donnell JM, Sumbilla C, Inesi G, Klein MG. Exogenous Ca2+-ATPase isoform effects on Ca2+□ transients of embryonic chicken and neonatal rat cardiac myocytes. *J Physiol* 528: 53–63, 2000.

Champion HC, Georgakopoulos D, Haldar S, Wang L, Wang Y, & Kass DA. Robust adenoviral and adeno-associated viral gene transfer to the in vivo murine heart, *Circulation,* 2003, 108, 2790-2797.

Chang KC, Schreur JH, Weiner MW, & Camacho SA. Impaired Ca2+ handling is an early manifestation of pressure-overload hypertrophy in rat hearts. Am J Physiol Heart Circ Physiol, Jul 1996; 271: H228 - H234. PMID: 8760179

Chen Y, Escoubet B, Prunier F, Amour J, Simonides WS, Vivien B, et al. Constitutive cardiac overexpression of sarcoplasmic/endoplasmic reticulum Ca2+-ATPase delays myocardial failure after myocardial infarction in rats at a cost of increased acute arrhythmias. Circulation 2004;109:1898–903.

Del Monte F, Butler K, Boecker W, Gwathmey JK, Hajjar RJ. Novel technique of aortic banding followed by gene transfer during hypertrophy and heart failure. *Physiol Genomics* 9: 49–56, 2002.

Del Monte F, Harding S, Schmidt U, Matsui T, Kang Z, William GD, Gwathmey JK, Rosenzweig A, Hajjar RJ. Restoration of contractile function in isolated cardiomyocytes from failing human hearts by gene transfer of SERCA2a. *Circulation* 100: 2308–2311, 1999.

Del Monte F, Williams E, Lebeche D, Schmidt U, Rosenzweig A, Gwathmey JK, Lewandowski ED, Hajjar RJ. Improvement in survival and cardiac metabolism after gene transfer of sarcoplasmic reticulum Ca2□-ATPase in a rat model of heart failure. *Circulation* 104: 1424–1429, 2001.

Dhu D et al. Direct comparison of efficiency and stability of gene transfer into the mammalian heart using adeno-associated virus versus adenovirus vectors. *J Thoracic Cardiovasc Surg.* 2003. 126(3); 671-679.

Du L et al. Differential myocardial gene delivery by recombinant serotype-specific adeno-associated viral vectors. Molecular Ther. 2004 10(3); 604-608.

Ding Z, Cach C, Sasse A, Godecke A, & Schrader J. A minimally invasive approach for efficient gene delivery to rodent hearts. *Gene Ther.* 2004; 11: 260-265.

Dode L, Carmeliet P, Dranias E, Herijgers P, Sipido KR, Raeymaekers L, Wuytack F. A SERCA2 pump with an increased Ca2□ affinity can lead to severe cardiac hypertrophy, stress intolerance and reduced life span. *J Mol Cell Cardiol* 41:308 –317, 2006.

Fromes Y, Salmon A, Wang X, et al. Gene delivery to the myocardium by intrapericardial injection. Gene Ther 1999; 6: 683-688.

Gilgenkrantz H et al. Transient expression of genes transferred in vivo into heart using first-generation adenoviral vectors: role of the immune response. *Hum Gene Ther.* 1995 Oct; 6(10): 1265-74.

Gregorevic P et al. Viral vectors for gene transfer to striated muscle. [Review] *Current Opinion in Molecul Therapeutics.* 2004. 6(5): 491-498.

Gregorevic P, Blankinship MJ, Allen JM, et al. Systemic delivery of genes to striated muscles using adeno-associated viral vectors. Nat Med 2004; 10: 828-834.

Guzman RJ, Lemarchand P, Crystal RG, Epstein SE, Finkel T. Efficient gene transfer into myocardium by direct injection of adenovirus vectors. Circ Res 1993; 73: 1202- 1207.

Gwathmey JK, Copelas L, MacKinnon R, Schoen FJ, Feldman MD, Grossman W, Morgan JP. Abnormal intracellular calcium handling in myocardium from patients with end-stage heart failure. *Circ Res* 61:701–76, 1987.

Gwathmey JK, Yerevanian AI, Hajjar RJ. Cardiac gene therapy with SERCA2a: from bench to bedside. J Mol Cell Cardiol 2011; 50: 803-812.

Hadri L, Bobe R, Kawase Y, et al. SERCA2a gene transfer enhances eNOS expression and activity in endothelial cells. Mol Ther 2010; 18: 1284-1292.

Hajjar RJ, U. Schmidt, T. Matsui, J. L. Guerrero, K. H. Lee, J. K. Gwathmey, G. W. Dec, M. J. Semigran, and A. Rosenzweig, Modulation of ventricular function through gene transfer in vivo. *Proc Natl Acad Sci.*, 1998, 95, 5251-5256.

Hajjar RJ, Zsebo K, Deckelbaum L, *et al.* Design of a phase 1/2 trial of intracoronary administration of AAV1/SERCA2a in patients with heart failure. J Card Fail 2008; 14: 355-367.

Hiranandani N, Raman S, Kalyanasundaram A, Periasamy M, Janssen PML. Frequency-dependent contractile strength in mice over- and underex- pressing the sarco(endo)plasmic reticulum calcium-ATPase. *Am J Physiol Regul Integr Comp Physiol* 293: R30–R36, 2007.

Hayase, M., Del Monte, F., Kawase, Y., Macneill, B.D., McGregor, J., Yoneyama, R., Hoshino, K., Tsuji, T., De Grand, A.M., Gwathmey, J.K., et al. (2005). Catheter-based antegrade intracoronary viral gene delivery with coronary venous blockade. Am J Physiol Heart Circ Physiol, Vol. 288, No. 6, (May 2005), pp. H2995-3000, ISSN 0363-6135

Hoshijima M, Ikeda Y, Iwanaga Y, et al. Chronic suppression of heart-failure progression by a pseudophosphorylated mutant of phospholamban via in vivo cardiac rAAV gene delivery. Nat Med 2002; 8: 864-871.

Huke S, Prasad V, Nieman ML, Nattamai KJ, Grupp IL, Lorenz JN, Periasamy M. Altered dose response to agonists in SERCA1-expressing hearts ex vivo and in vivo. *Am J Physiol Heart Circ Physiol* 283: H958 –H966, 2002.

Ikeda Y, Gu Y, Iwanaga Y, Hoshijima M, Oh SS, Giordano FJ, Chen J, Nigro V, Peterson KL, Chien KR, & Ross J. Restoration of deficient membrane proteins in the cardiomyopathic hamster by in vivo cardiac gene transfer. *Circulation,* 2002, 105, 502-508.

Inagaki K, Fuess S, Storm TA, et al. Robust systemic transduction with AAV9 vectors in mice: efficient global cardiac gene transfer superior to that of AAV8. Mol Ther 2006; 14: 45-53.

Iwatate M, Gu Y, Dieterle T, Iwanaga Y, Peterson KL, Hoshijima M, Chien KR, & Ross J, In vivo high-efficiency transcoronary gene delivery and Cre-LoxP gene switching in the adult mouse heart, *Gene Therapy,* 2003, 10(21), 1814-1820.

Jaski BE, Jessup ML, Mancini DM, *et al.* Calcium upregulation by percutaneous administration of gene therapy in cardiac disease (CUPID Trial), a first-in-human phase 1/2 clinical trial. J Card Fail 2009; 15: 171-181.

Janssen PM, Stull LB, Marban E. Myofilament properties comprise the rate-limiting step for cardiac relaxation at body temperature in the rat. *Am J Physiol Heart Circ Physiol* 282: H499–H507, 2002.

Janssen PML, Periasamy M. Determinants of frequency-dependent con- traction and relaxation of mammalian myocardium. *J Mol Cell Cardiol* 43: 523–531, 2007.

Jessup M, Greenberg B, Mancine D, Cappola T, Pauly DF, Jaski B, Yaroshinsky A, Zsebo KM, Dittrich H, Hajjar RJ; Calcium upregulation by percutaneous administration of gene therapy in cardiac disease (CUPID): a phase 2 trial of intracoronary gene therapy of sarcoplasmic reticulum Ca2+-ATPase in patients with advanced hear failure. Circ 124(3):304-313, 2011.

Kaspar BK, Roth DM, Lai NC, et al. Myocardial gene transfer and long-term expression following intracoronary delivery of adeno-associated virus. J Gene Med 2005; 7: 316-324.

Kass-Eisler A, Falck-Pedersen E, Alvira M, et al. Quantitative determination of adenovirus-mediated gene delivery to rat cardiac myocytes in vitro and in vivo. Proc Natl Acad Sci U S A 1993; 90: 11498-11502.

Kawamoto S, et al. Widespread and early myocardial gene expression by adeno-associated virus vector type 6 with a beta-actin hybrid promoter. *Molecular Ther.* 2005. 11(6); 980-985.

Kaye, D.M., Preovolos, A., Marshall, T., Byrne, M., Hoshijima, M., Hajjar, R., Mariani, J.A., Pepe, S., Chien, K.R. & Power, J.M. (2007). Percutaneous cardiac recirculation-mediated gene transfer of an inhibitory phospholamban peptide reverses advanced heart failure in large animals. J Am Coll Cardiol, Vol. 50, No. 3, (July 2007), pp. 253-260, ISSN 1558-3597

Kotin RM. Large-scale recombinant adeno-associated virus production. Human Mole Gene. 20(1) R2-R6, 2011.

Lalli MJ, Yong J, Prasad V, Hashimoto K, Plank D, Babu GJ, Kirkpatrick D, Walsh RA, Sussman M, Yatani A, Marban E, Peria- samy M. Sarcoplasmic reticulum Ca2□ ATPase (SERCA1) 1a-structurally substitutes for SERCA2a in the cardiac sarcoplasmic reticulum and in- creases cardiac Ca2□ handling capacity. *Circ Res* 89: 160–167, 2001.

Loukianov E, Ji Y, Grupp IL, Kirkpatrick DL, Baker DL, Louki- anova T, Grupp G, Lytton J, Walsh RA, Periasamy M. Enhanced myocardial contractility and increased Ca2□ transport function in transgenic hearts expressing the fast-twitch skeletal muscle sarcoplasmic reticulum Ca2+-ATPase. *Circ Res* 83: 889–897, 1998.

MacGowan GA. The myofilament force-calcium relationship as a target for positive inotropic therapy in congestive heart failure. *Cardiovasc Drugs Ther* 19: 203–210, 2005.

Maurice JP, Hata JA, Shah AS, et al. Enhancement of cardiac function after adenoviral-mediated in vivo intracoronary beta2-adrenergic receptor gene delivery. J Clin Invest 1999; 104: 21-29.

Marston SB, de Tombe PP. Troponin phosphorylation and myofilament Ca2+ sensitivity in heart failure: increased or decreased? J Mol Cell Cardiol. 2008 Nov;45(5):603-7. Epub 2008 Jul 19.

Miyamoto MI, del Monte F, Schmidt U, DiSalvo TS, Kang ZB, Matsui T, Guerrero JL, Gwathmey JK, Rosenzweig A, Hajjar RJ. Adenoviral gene transfer of SERCA2a improves left-ventricular function in aortic- banded rats in transition to heart failure. *Proc Natl Acad Sci USA* 97: 793–798, 2000.

O'Donnell JM, Pound K., Xu X, and Lewandowski ED. SERCA1 Expression enhances the metabolic efficiency of improved contractility in post ischemic hearts. *J Mol Cell Cardio, 47(5):614-21,2009.*

O'Donnell JM, Fields A, Xu X, Chowdhury SA, Geenen DL, and J Bi. Limited functional and metabolic improvements in hypertrophic and healthy hearts expressing the skeletal muscle isoform of SERCA1 by adenoviral gene transfer in vivo. *Amer J Physiol (Heart and Circ.)* 295(6):H2483-94, 2008. PMID 18952713

O'Donnell JM, and ED Lewandowski. Efficient, Cardiac-Specific Adenoviral Gene Transfer by Isolated Retrograde Perfusion *In Vivo. Gene Therapy* 12, 958-964, 2005. PMID15789062

O'Donnell JM and ED Lewandowski. Controlling specificity and efficiency of adenoviral gene transfer in heart by catheter based coronary perfusion. In: Gene Therapy Prospective assessment in its societal context. Niewohner J. & Tannert C. (Eds), Amsterdam, Netherlands, Elsevier (pub) 2006, p.33-46.

O'Donnell JM, Sumbilla C, Hailun M, Farrance I, Cavagna M, Klein M, Inesi G. Tight control of exogenous SERCA expression is required to obtain acceleration of calcium transients with minimal cytotoxic effect in cardiac myocytes. *Circ Res* 88: 415–421, 2001.

Perez NG, Hashimoto K, McCune S, Altschuld RA, Marban E. Origin of contractile dysfunction in heart failure: calcium cycling versus myo- filaments. *Circulation* 99: 1077–1083, 1999.

Periasamy M, Huke S. SERCA pump level is a critical determinant of Ca2□ homeostasis and cardiac contractility. *J Mol Cell Cardiol* 33:1053–1063, 2001.

Pinz, I., Tian, R., Belke, D., Swanson, E., Dillmann, W. & Ingwall, J.S. (2011). Compromised myocardial energetics in hypertrophied mouse hearts diminish the beneficial effect of overexpressing SERCA2A. J Biol Chem, Vol., No., (February 2011), ISSN 1083-351X

Prasad KMR. Xu Y., Yang Z., Acton ST., French BA. Robust cardiomyocyte-specific gene expression following systemic injection of AAV: In vivo gene delivery follows a poisson distribution. Gene Therapy 19(1): 43-52; 2011.

Raake PW, Hinkel R, Muller S, et al. Cardio-specific long-term gene expression in a porcine model after selective pressure-regulated retroinfusion of adeno-associated viral (AAV) vectors. Gene Ther 2008; 15: 12-17.

Reyes-Juarez JL, & Zarain-Herzberg A. Gene therapy in cardiovascular disease. In Gene Therapy Applications. InTech. 95-126, 2011

Sipido KR, Bangheluwe P. Targeting sarcoplasmic reticulum Ca2+ uptake to improve heart failure: hit or miss. Circ Res. 2010 106(2):230-233. PMID 20133907

Stratford-Perricaudet LD, Makeh I, Perricaudet M, Briand P. Widespread long-term gene transfer to mouse skeletal muscles and heart. J Clin Invest 1992; 90: 626-630.

Su H, Lu R, Kan YW. Adeno-associated viral vector-mediated vascular endothelial growth factor gene transfer induces neovascular formation in ischemic heart. Proceedings of the National Academy of Sciences of the United States of America 2000;97(25):13801–6. [PubMed: 11095751]

Su H, et al. Adeno-associated viral vector delivers cardiac-specific and hypoxia-inducible VEGF expression in ischemic mouse hearts. *Proc Natl Acad Sci.* 2004 101(46): 16280-16285.

Svensson EC, Marshall DJ, Woodard K, Lin H, Jiang F, Chu L, et al. Efficient and stable transduction of cardiomyocytes after intramyocardial injection or intracoronary perfusion with recombinant adeno-associated virus vectors. Circulation 1999;99(2):201–5. [PubMed: 9892583]

Talukder MAH, Kalyanasundaram A, Zhao X, Zuo L, Bhupathy P, Babu GJ, et al. Expression of SERCA isoform with faster Ca2+ transport properties improves postischemic cardiac function and Ca2+ handling and decreases myocardial infarction. Am J Physiol Heart Circ Physiol 2007;293:H2418–28.

Teucher N, Prestle J, Seidler T, Currie S, Elliott EB, Reynolds DR, Schott P, Wagner S, Kogler H, Inesi G, Bers DM, Hasenfuss G, Smith GL. Excessive sarcoplasmic/endoplasmic reticulum Ca2□-ATPase expression causes increased sarcoplasmic reticulum Ca2□ uptake but decreases myocyte shortening. *Circulation* 110: 3553–3559, 2004.

Vangheluwe P, Tjwa M, Van Den Bergh A, Louch WE, Beullens M,

Wang Z, Zhu T, Qiao C, Zhou L, Wang B, Zhang J, Chen C, Li J, Xiao X. Adeno-associated virus serotype 8 efficiently dlivers genes to muscle and heart. Nat Biotechnol. 2005 Mar;23(3):321-8. Epub 2005 Feb 27.

Wasala, NB., Shin JH., Duan D. The evolution of heart gene delivery vectors. J Gene Med. 13(10);557-65, 2011.

Weisser-Thomas J, Dieterich E, Janssen PML, Schmidt-Schweda S, Maier LS, Sumbilla C, Pieske B. Method-related effects of adenovirus- mediated LacZ and SERCA1 gene transfer on contractile behavior of cultured failing human cardiomyocytes. *J Pharm Tox Meth* 51: 91–103, 2005. PMID: 15767202

White, J.D., Thesier, D.M., Swain, J.B.D., Katz, M.G., Tomasulo, C., Henderson, A., Wang, L., Yarnall, C., Fargnoli, A., Sumaroka, M., et al. (2011). Myocardial gene delivery using molecular cardiac surgery with recombinant adeno-associated virus vectors in vivo. Gene Therapy, Vol., No., pp. 1-7

Wright MJ, Rosenthal E, Stewart L, Wightman LML, Miller AD, Latchman DS, Marber MS. Galactosidase staining following intra-coronary infusion of cationic liposomes in the in vivo rabbit heart is produced by microinfarction rather than effective gene transfer: a caution- ary tale. *Gene Ther* 5: 301–308, 1998.

M. J. Wright, L. M. L. Wightman, D. S. Latchman, and M. S. Marber, In vivo myocardial gene transfer: optimization and evaluation of intracoronary gene delivery in vivo, *Gene Therapy,* 2001, 8, 1833-1839.

Xie, Q., et al. The atomic structure of adeno-associated virus (AAV-2), a vector for human gene therapy. *Proc Natl Acad Sci.* 2002. 99: 10405-10410.

Yue Y, Ghosh A, Long C, et al. A single intravenous injection of adeno-associated virus serotype-9 leads to whole body skeletal muscle transduction in dogs. Mol Ther 2008; 16: 1944-1952

Zhu T, et al. Sustained whole-body functional rescue in congestive heart failure and muscular dystrophy hamsters by systemic gene transfer. *Circ.* 2005. 112(17): 2650-2690.